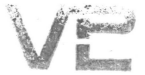

ESSENTIAL

YOGA

ESSENTIAL

YOGA

SARAH HERRINGTON

First published in the USA in 2013 by
Fair Winds Press, a member of
Quayside Publishing Group
100 Cummings Center
Suite 406-L
Beverly, MA 01915-6101
www.fairwindspress.com

17 16 15 14 13   1 2 3 4 5

ISBN: 978-159233-553-4

Digital edition published in 2013
eISBN: 978-1-61058-742-6

Library of Congress-in-Publication Data available

All photographs by Jonathan Conklin Photography with the exception of the following, shutterstock.com:
front cover; 12 (left); 14 (upper left); 21; 42; 58; 74; 90; 106, 122
Kotaro Kawashima, 140; 160 (top)
Back cover, Lasonic Sivongxay

Created by Moseley Road Inc.
Editor: Erica Gordon-Mallin
Designer: Danielle Scaramuzzo
Cover Design: Gus Yoo
Template Designer: Lisa Purcell
Photographer: Jonathan Conklin Photography, Inc.
Models: Sara Blowers, Sarah Herrington, and James W. White

CONTENTS

CONTENTS

CONTENTS

I. YOGA RIGHT NOW

Yoga is an amazing practice. Exercising the mind, body, and spirit, it benefits everyone, regardless of body type, physical ability, mental ability, age, background, or income. In fact, anyone who can breathe can do yoga and feel the effects of growing calmer and stronger in body and mind.

Yoga means "yoke" in Sanskrit, an ancient language from India, and accordingly yoga is a practice that brings together the body, mind, and spirit. In the yoga tradition, it's believed that we cannot touch one of the three without affecting the other; when we practice the physical poses, we are also training our minds and elevating our spirits. Along with lean, powerful muscles, a tight, toned physique, better flexibility, and increased strength, yoga will also bring about focus and energy. It will calm your mind, lift your mood, and even improve your connection to your spirit as it transforms your body. In short, yoga will get you into shape from the inside out.

All too often, people think of yoga as a slow practice that must be learned with great patience and intuition…over a long, long period of time. After all, the 14th *sutra* in the *Yoga Sutras*, a classical text written down by Patanjali, tells us, "Practice becomes firmly rooted when well attended to for a long time, without break and in all earnestness."

But yoga also has a place in the lives of busy people. While patience and seriousness have their roles, yoga is above all a joyful practice. If you think your day is too jam-packed for yoga, or if you believe you need to buy (or even be) something before you start, think again: there is no reason not to make yoga a part of your daily life, right now.

WHY ESSENTIAL YOGA?

This book is not about meeting a requirement, going through the motions, or ticking a checklist for "perfect" yoga form. Instead, these lessons give you the tools to make yoga part of your mind and body. No matter how pressed for time you may be, yoga can benefit you right at this moment.

The spirit of Essential Yoga can be summed up in a word: "now." In Sanskrit, this is translated as *atha*, which happens to be the very first word in the *Yoga Sutras*. This book is meant to inspire you and give you tools you can

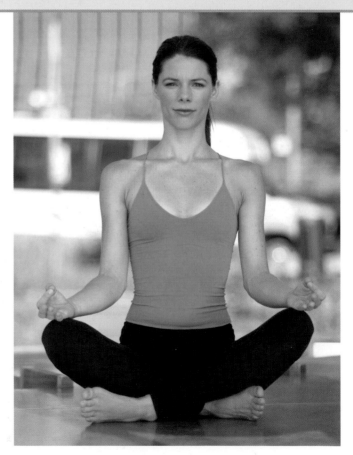

use right now. There is no reason to wait to learn about yoga breathing, meditation, and concentration, and yoga poses that will help your body grow strong and healthy and flexible. There is no reason to wait for inspiration!

If you are nervous about starting yoga or it is totally new to you, don't worry. In fact, you can bring your nervousness or skepticism to the mat. Yoga is never about denying what you feel, but getting to know what you feel. You will learn where your body is tight (in your hips, or hamstrings). You will learn where you are nervous (maybe arm balances make you sweat). You will learn what you love (the ultra-relaxing Corpse Pose might be your favorite thing ever). The point is that you can act with full aware

ness of your feelings and bring them along with you.

Armed with the information in this book, nothing should stop you from doing yoga. You don't need to be flexible, nor must you be physically strong. You don't have to have a lot of free time to practice each day, or the inclination to read about the history of the practice.

While the tradition of yoga is vast, deep, wide, the point of entry is always found in the word "now." A small but profound example of this lies in the breath. If you get distracted in a yoga pose, or in life, you can tune into the inhale or exhale happening now. This will bring you back to the present moment, where the tradition of yoga is very much alive. So let's get started!

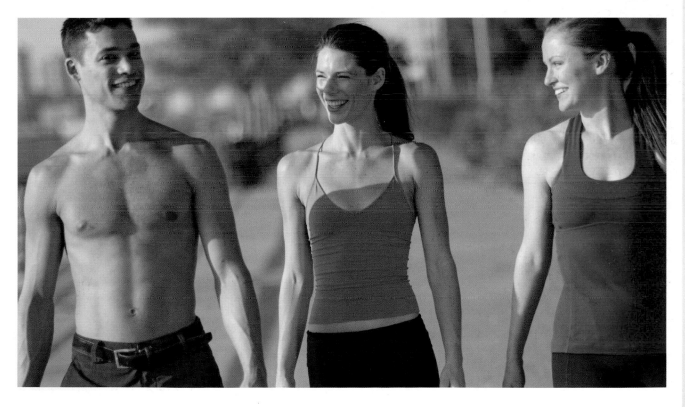

MAXIMIZING YOUR TIME

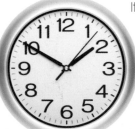

If you have never even rolled out a yoga mat, then perfect: This book will guide you, step by step, through the essentials of yoga. If you are an intermediate or advanced practitioner, this book is for you too; filled with poses at many different levels, plus many variations. This course will challenge you.

To maximize your time during yoga practice, set an intention. Do you want to trim your waistline, or simply work on touching your toes? If you are seeking energy, check out the Fire Up section; if you are looking to calm down, you may want to look at Moonlight Wind-Down. If you want to understand the poses and sequencing that occurs in a studio yoga class make sure you try the Sun Salutations and read How to Ace a Studio Class (page 138). Of course, I hope you will read the whole book. This course can be followed straight through, start to finish, as well as dipped into now and then.

Although you may think you need lots of time for yoga, carrying out just a couple of poses after rolling out of bed or a breathing exercise on your lunch break can make an immense difference in your day.

WHAT YOU REALLY NEED
(AND WHAT YOU DON'T)

In yoga practice, you really need an open mind and a willingness to try. Yogis don't use the word "practice" for nothing. Yoga is about trying, making mistakes, and learning; the sincerity of your interest is what matters.

Although you may often see yogis with focused expressions on their faces, I assure you: they are also having fun. Yoga is profound play. It is experimentation. In yoga, you experience a balance of effort and ease. It is your willingness to try yoga that will bring you benefits,

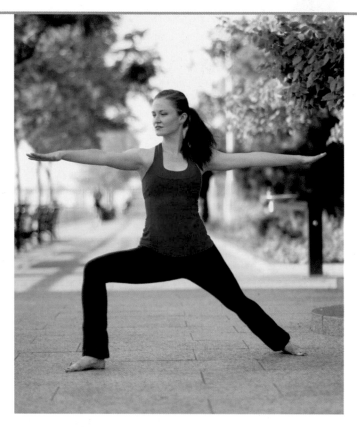

both immediately and over time. While you have to work hard in some ways (for example, it can be hard to balance), yoga is also joyous.

What you don't need in yoga is perfection: yoga is more about your individual journey than arriving at "perfect" form. While we will review the form of the different poses and shapes in this book, they are meant as guidelines. Everybody is different. Just because your Tree Pose looks different than the one in the book doesn't mean you are not doing it "correctly." Yoga is about the spirit of the poses as well as the shapes. If you feel like a Warrior (strong, grounded, and focused), chances are you're "doing it right"—even if your Warrior III may not look exactly like the one on page 67.

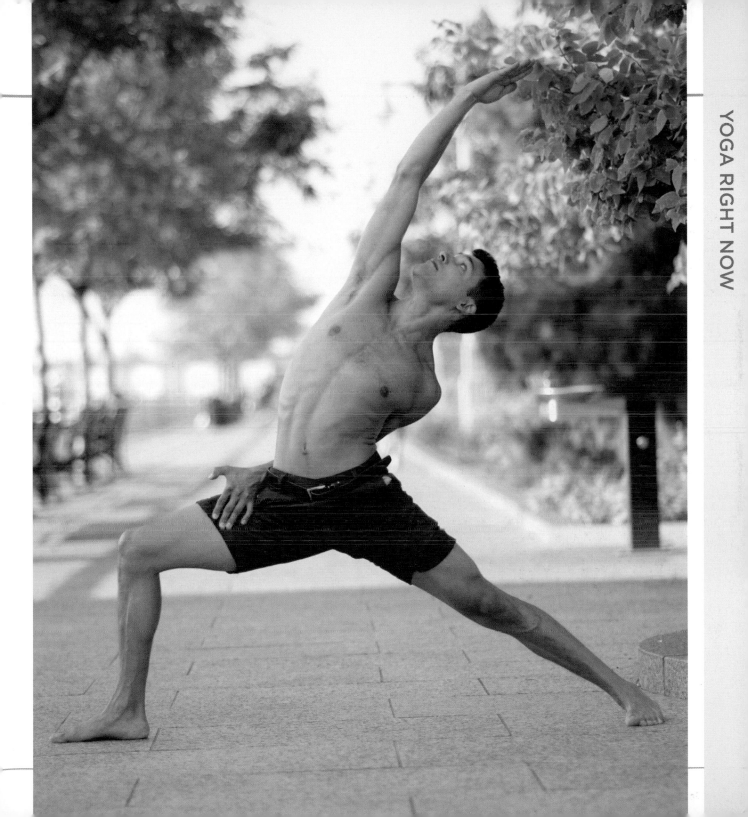

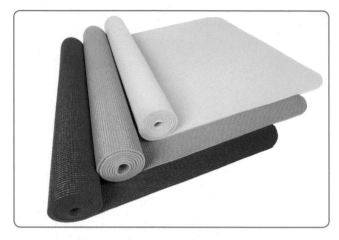

Although you don't need many material objects in order to practice yoga, some are of benefit. It is beneficial to have a yoga mat to practice on. Yoga mats are made from a sticky, rubbery material and provide traction for the body. They help to keep you from falling. And if you do fall over, there's a nice squishy surface to land on.

Yoga mats also delineate space. You'll find this especially helpful if you venture out into a yoga class. This way, you know where to line up your Warrior I and your neighbor will know to do the same.

And yoga mats have a trick: they often absorb sweat. This is wonderful because even though some poses may look deceptively simple, they can really get your heart pumping! Remember that sweat is your body's way of detoxifying and cooling. If you sweat in practice, that's normal; if you don't, that's all right too. What's more, if you don't have a yoga mat at this time, don't let that stop you. I really mean it when I say all you need for yoga is your body and your breath.

It's great to have stretchy yoga clothes, too, but if you don't have them, start anyway. It's also wonderful to have a designated yoga spot in your home which signifies yoga time for you. Keep this place free of clutter to help keep your mind clear and allow you space to stretch out. But if you do not have a yoga space at this time, again, start anyway: the magic of yoga lies in beginning it.

Many ancient yogis believed the yoga poses and breathing exercises described this book to be natural to the human body. It is as if these poses and exercises are already within you, waiting to come out. If you watch a child, you may see him or her naturally trying some of these poses. For example, when children learn to walk they often begin the exploration by propping themselves up in Downward-Facing Dog. There is even a pose called Happy Baby, and we've all seen babies take on this pose naturally (and yes, looking quite cheery while doing it). So while it may seem strange at first to try some of these shapes, they are somewhat natural shapes for your body to be in. With time you will get used to them, and hopefully feel happy and healthy—growing ever more so!—in all of them.

VOCABULARY LESSON

Here is a list of terms and phrases you may find useful during this course.

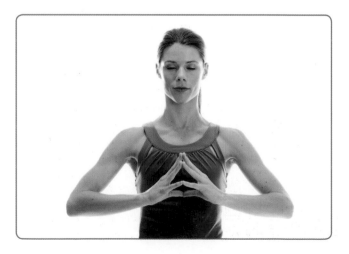

heart-center

We sometimes use this term to indicate the front of the chest. Often, we bring our hands to meet here when we center ourselves or assume a twisting position. Heart-center is felt to be a place of energy and emotion. For example, many yoga poses ask us to dip our head below the heart-center in a symbolic gesture to lead life from the heart, not just the head.

tuck your tailbone

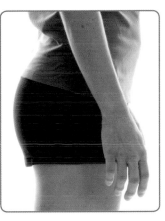

At some points in the following pages you may be asked to "tuck your tailbone." You can also think of this as pulling the navel toward the spine. Often we unconsciously have a deep sway in our lower backs, allowing our bellies and bottoms to stick out. This instruction is not about vanity or coming into a certain look, but rather an issue of alignment and protecting the spine. Also, tucking the tailbone often engages the core.

core

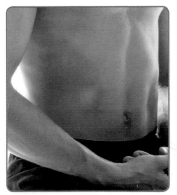

Yogis often talk about the core, referring to the group of muscles at the center of the body, including the abdominal muscles, gluteal muscles, and back. Strengthening the core is very important in yoga. A strong core protects the back. All yoga poses radiate from

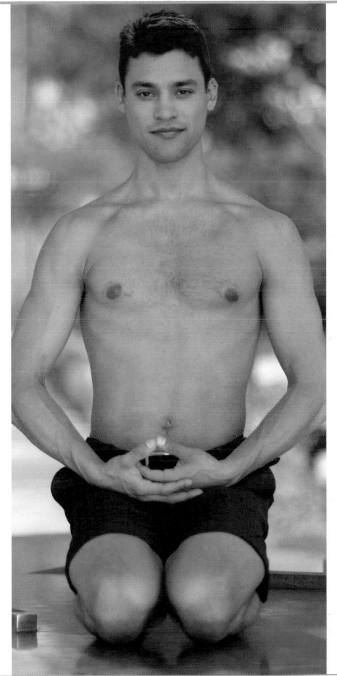

the body's center, so taking the time to make the core strong affects the integrity of all poses. Core strengthening can be symbolic, too: having a strong inner core means drawing on strength from the inside before reaching outward.

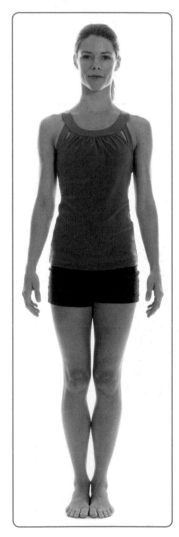

root down to rise up

Sometimes yoga teachers use this phrase, reminding students to feel the strength of their connection to the ground. The phrase is about taking time to set up the foundation of a pose before rising up into its full expression. For instance, in Warriors I, II, and III, you will take the time to find a strong foundation before moving into the arm and head positions. Once you feel grounded in a pose, you can begin to shine and dance.

neutral spine

At some points in the course, you'll be asked to to adopt a neutral spine. Think of your spine as an energy cord that runs up and down your body, from the base of your torso to your head. While in some poses you may sway this cord from side to side, or tuck the tail of it (your

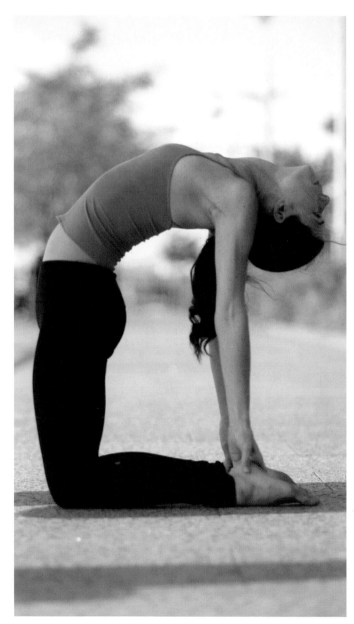

tailbone) under, in other poses you'll find it's best to let your spine stay as neutral as possible: neither arched nor hunched.

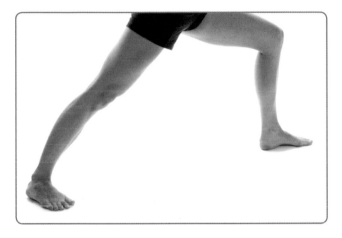

heel-to-heel alignment

In some standing postures, such as the Warrior poses, you will be asked to focus on heel-to-heel alignment. This simply means that if you look at the position of your feet, you should be able to draw a straight imaginary line from the heel of your front foot to the heel of your back foot. Conversely, you may like a more narrow stance, where you'll be able to draw a straight imaginary line from the heel of your front foot to the inside arch of your back foot.

reaching from, not to

This concept is connected to the ideas of strengthening the core and rooting down to rise up. The idea is to come into integration in a pose before reaching outward. Even when your arms are extended in a Warrior pose, try thinking of the reach coming from deep within yourself, rather than grasping for something external.

Your gaze can also "reach"; it is important to notice where you are looking while performing a pose. The idea is not to look for something outside of yourself, but to let your gaze be soft, truly originating from within. In general, although the poses and movements of yoga might look beautiful, the real action of yoga is coming from within. The intention of movement is more important than the actual reaching. This phrase is about taking time to orient your body, breath, and mind from within before reaching for something outside yourself.

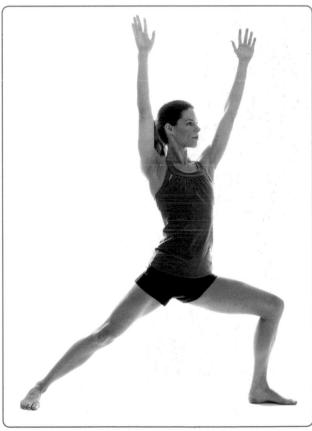

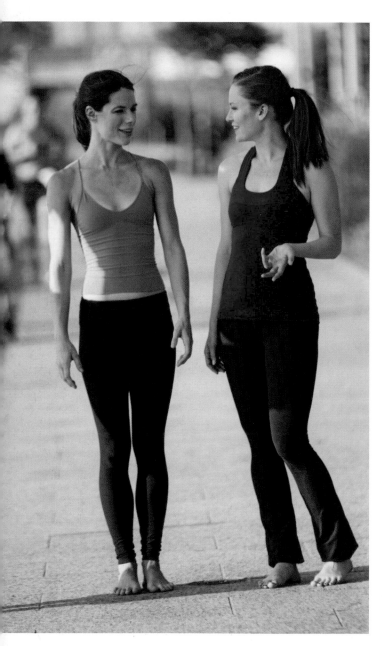

SCHOOLS OF YOGA

If you enter a yoga studio or pick up a magazine, DVD, or book on yoga, you will likely be confronted with many different styles and techniques, most with Sanskrit names. It can be a confounding to see so many different names, and even more confounding to talk to diehard devotees of one style who never try any of the others. All styles hold immense benefits for the body and mind. (The style we'll draw upon in the following pages is, for the most part, Hatha Vinyasa, with a little Power yoga thrown in.) Here are some of the most common schools of yoga.

ASHTANGA YOGA

Ashtanga is an active, athletic style of yoga. Through Ashtanga, you work toward synchronizing breath with movement through performing a progressive series of postures. This style was originally devised to help teenage boys in India to utilize extra energy and redirect their active minds to prepare for meditation. Master teacher Pattabhi Jois is to thank for bringing Ashtanga yoga to the United States in the 1970s. "Mysore Style" Ashtanga (referring to Mysore, India) is a supervised self-led practice in which everyone moves at his or her own level.

BHAKTI YOGA

Also known as Devotional yoga, Bhakti emphasizes chanting, or *kirtan*, and storytelling as ways to express and explore spiritual devotion. Kirtan music is typically very uplifting, even for those who do not understand the Sanskrit lyrics.

BIKRAM YOGA

Bikram is practiced in a room heated to 105°F (40°C). In each Bikram class or practice, the same series of twenty-six postures are carried out.

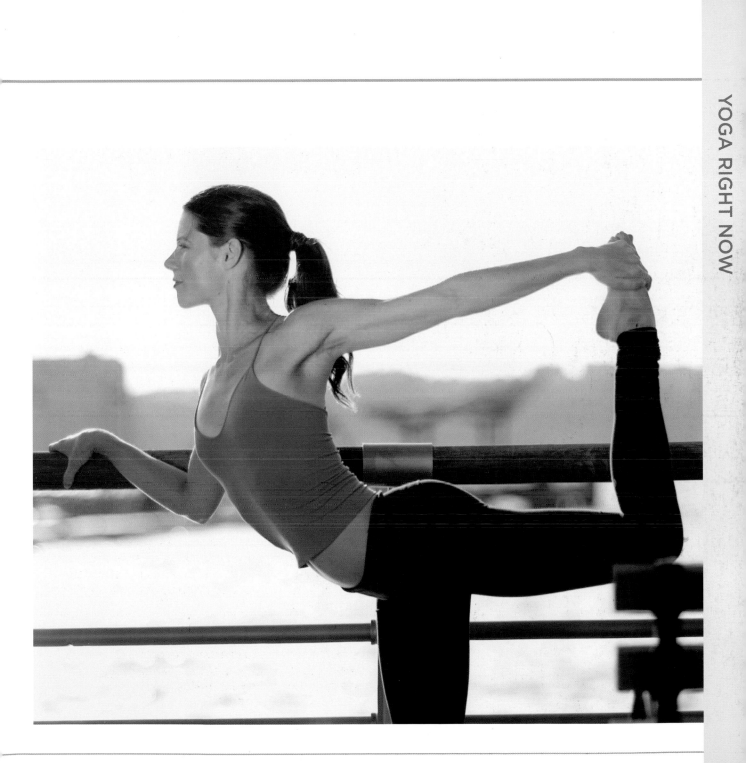

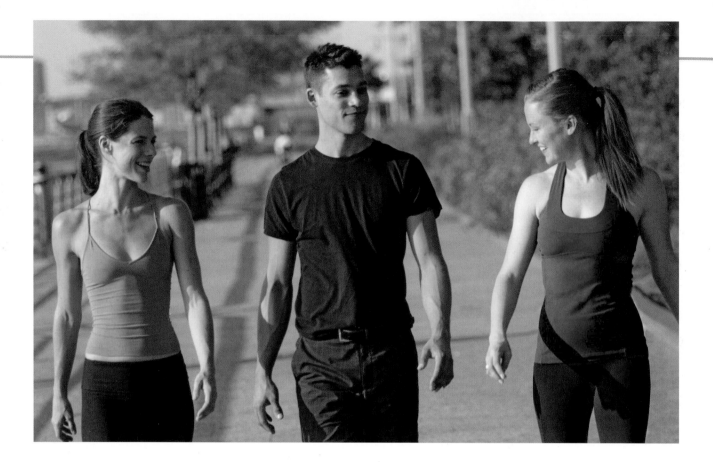

HATHA YOGA

Hatha is the foundation of many yoga styles. It incorporates poses, *pranayama* (breathing techniques), and meditation to cultivate an even state of mind, a well body, and reduced stress. The word *hatha* suggests balance; *ha* and *tha* mean "sun" and "moon" respectively. Hatha yoga can be relaxing on its own, or it can form a foundation for more rigorous practice.

IYENGAR YOGA

Developed by master teacher B. K. S. Iyengar, this style focuses on precise alignment and often incorporates props like cushions, blankets, straps, and blocks.

In Iyengar, you often hold poses longer than you would in other styles. With its slow pace and use of props, it was developed to heal physical ailments and can be great for physical therapy.

JIVAMUKTI YOGA

Founded by teachers Sharon Gannon and David Life in New York City in the 1980s, Jivamukti is a vigorous practice incorporating a steady flow of poses with chanting and breath work. In this style, Vinyasa yoga is combined with spiritual elements like meditation and devotion, along with an emphasis on nonviolence.

KIDS YOGA

Kids yoga introduces children and teens to yoga practice in ways that are developmentally appropriate. The term encompasses yoga for a wide range of ages, from birth through teen (when practitioners can begin adult class). Often storytelling and song are used to explore yoga in a way that is educational and fun.

KUNDALINI YOGA

Kundalini focuses on awakening energy at the base of the spine and drawing it upward. Breathing exercises, chanting, meditation and an introspective investigation of poses, along with repetitive cycles of practice, help to awaken energy in this tradition.

POWER YOGA

Power yoga is a largely Western interpretation of Ashtanga, bringing an emphasis on strength and meditative breathing into the practice. Poses flow from one to the next and are often held for some time, allowing the body to create heat and sweat. The goal is a strong body and clear mind, combining intensity with deep relaxation.

PRENATAL YOGA

Prenatal yoga serves the expectant mother. Breath work and physical poses are designed for the woman's changing body and her needs during pregnancy.

VINYASA YOGA

Sometimes referred to as Vinyasa Flow, this style aligns breath with movement, resulting in a dynamic flow. Often poses are held for just one to five breaths, making this an active and often expressive style of yoga. Emphasis is placed on breath and the journey in between poses as well as the poses themselves. This is a popular style in the West and can include creative sequences that keep you moving.

SANSKRIT CHEAT SHEET

Sanskrit is an ancient language from India, where yoga has its roots. Many of the poses in this book have Sanskrit names, which are listed under their English names.

One word you'll hear a lot in yoga classes is *asana*, which translates literally to "seat." Accordingly, in yoga we are supposed to find a comfortable spot, or "seat," in all of the poses we assume, so that we feel steady and at ease. In common usage, the word *asana* has come to mean "pose." Put simply, an *asana* is a yoga pose.

You'll find the word *asana* inside many of the pose names in this book. For example, Tadasana means Mountain Pose and Savasana means Corpse Pose, also known as Rest Pose.

Here is a short list of other Sanskrit terms you may encounter in the following pages or in yoga classes.

drishti: a gazing point for a pose. When you practice Dancer's Pose, for example, it helps to find your *drishti*.

mantra: a phrase that is repeated in the mind.

mudra: a yogic hand position.

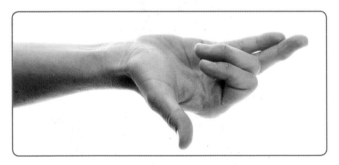

namaste: translates to "The light in me honors the light in you." It's a nice way to greet people and say "thank you" in yoga class. It is signaled by bringing the hands together in front of the heart.

OM: a universal and primal sound. Singing OM brings a soothing and unifying vibration to the body and mind; at the beginning of a yoga class, it indicates the beginning of collective effort through collecting voices into one note. It also signifies the intention of connecting to goodness, to a source.

pranayama: refers to yogic breathing exercises. Changing our breathing can change how we feel. We can get more energy by breathing in certain ways, or relax our energy by breathing in other ways.

savasana: translates to "corpse" (*sava*) "seat" or "pose" (*asana*). Taken literally, Savasana or Corpse Pose evokes the process of dying—or, a bit less morbidly, the process of letting go and surrendering to complete relaxation.

SOME MANTRAS TO TRY:

- Let go
- I am happy, I am free
- May I be happy
- *Lokah samastah sukhino bhavantu:* May all beings everywhere be happy and free.

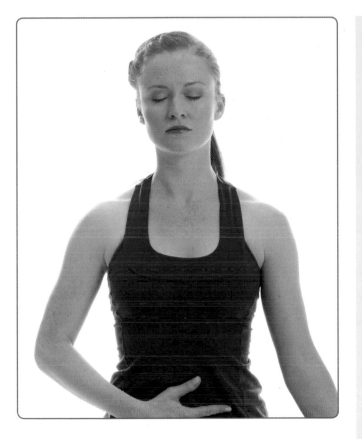

CHIN MUDRA

One very common yogic hand position is Chin Mudra, in which the thumb lightly covers the forefinger/pointer finger and the rest of the fingers remain extended. The pose is symbolic: the thumb represents the universe, the finger the individual. By taking this shape we remind ourselves that we are not alone; we are part of the universe, and the universe is helping us. It also signifies a connection of energy, looping it back around so none is lost.

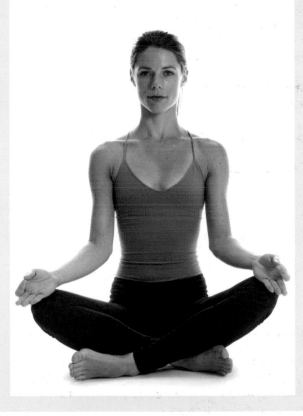

ujjayi: translates to victorious breath"—a special way of breathing through the nose with the mouth closed, so that breath resonates in the back of the throat. Ujjayi breath makes a sound evocative of the ocean. Combined with flowing *vinyasa*, *ujjayi* creates internal head, leading to purification of the body.

vinyasa: translates to "in an ordered sequence" (*vi*) + "on purpose or with intention" (*nyasa*). The term describes movements carried out conscientiously, in a flowing sequence.

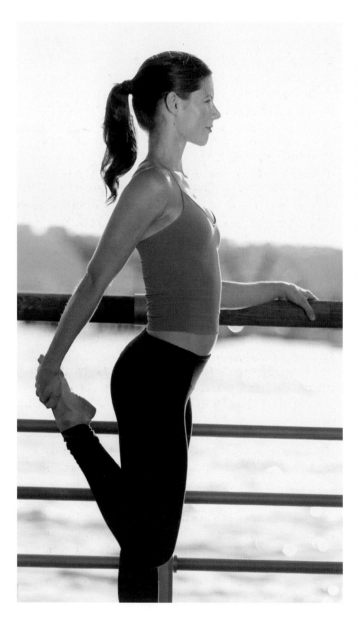

BREATHING BASICS

In yoga, breath is thought to serve as a link between the mind and the body. Bringing awareness to our breath strengthens that link. Focusing on breathing also helps to reinforce our connection with the present moment. That's the great thing about breath: it's always happening, now. You can't really hold onto it forever; you have to practice letting go. There is always a fresh in-breath after every out-breath. The very act of breathing itself is a gesture of giving and receiving. Yoga reminds us of the gift our breath gives us, and the power of this gift.

If we change how we breathe, we can truly change how we feel. The link between body and mind through breath is apparent when you think about it. When we are tired our breath may change to a yawn, or slow sluggish breathing. When we are frightened we make take short sharp breaths, breathing shallowly from the

AVOIDING DISTRACTION

You may find that distractions arise. Perhaps something in your physical body, such as an itch, the urge to move, or some sudden tension, will demand attention. Your mind may also pull you away as you think about your to-do list or wonder which emails you may be missing. It can be very challenging to keep your awareness on even a few breaths, so much so that performing five fully focused inhales and exhales can be a feat!

When you notice that your attention is wandering, don't feel bad about it. Instead, understand that that this is part of the process of mindful breathing. That moment when you realize you've been thinking is actually a moment of "waking up." Try silently labeling it as "thinking," and then come back to your breath.

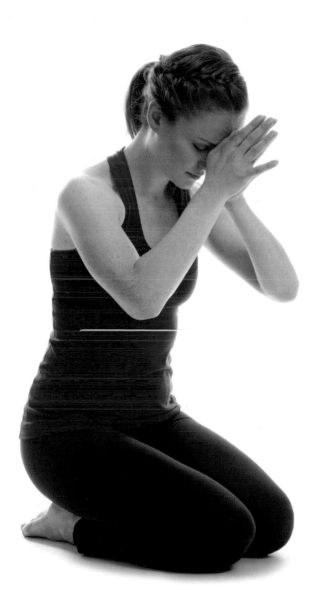

POSITIONING YOURSELF

When practicing any breathing technique, the first step is to get comfortable. Your body should be stable and strong, yet full of ease so you can then bring attention to the mind and breath. You can try sitting cross-legged on the floor, or even in Full Lotus Pose (see page 120). It is nice to sit on half of a cushion or pillow, to allow your hips to rest above your knees. With some gentle propping up, your spine can rest straighter and the front of your body will be more open, leading to a broader chest and more space in the lungs, which in turn facilitates clearer, fuller breathing.

chest. In yoga practice we like to reverse this cause and response. Instead of just letting our natural emotions and thoughts change breath, we can use our breath to change emotional and mental states.

In general, when you work to slow down the breath you calm the mind and nervous system. Focusing on the exhale, and making the exhale longer than the inhale, can also calm the mind. When you speed up the breath, you bring energy into the mind and body. When you work to make the breath even, with inhalations and exhalations of roughly the same duration, your thoughts and emotions can also become more balanced.

When practicing breathing techniques, sit as tall as you can possibly sit without straining. The idea is to allow your lungs to expand to full capacity, to give the full amount of space to the front of your body. By sitting up tall, the back of your body can thoroughly support you.

The following breathing techniques can be practiced both on the yoga mat and in daily life.

UJJAYI BREATH

Ujjayi breath is commonly used throughout Vinyasa classes, where one pose flows into the other. This technique is audible; listening to the inhales and exhales can help to guide your movements.

Some people describe Ujjayi breath as the sound of the ocean waves, or the sound of Darth Vader breathing. Inhales are taken through the nose and exhales pool in the back of the throat, the upper back of the palate.

When trying Ujjayi for the first time, keep your mouth open. Hold your hand in front of your mouth as if it were a mirror. Inhale through your nose, then exhale out an open mouth onto your imaginary mirror, as if you were fogging it up with your breath. Try this a few times, using the exhale to heat up and fog your "hand-mirror."

Then, try making the same sound and action with your lips lightly sealed. See if you can hear your breath, even as your mouth stays shut. The sound may be less strongly audible, but it is there.

Ujjayi breath is highly warming, helping to create heat in the body as you move and stretch. It is also deeply calming, giving you a point of mental focus.

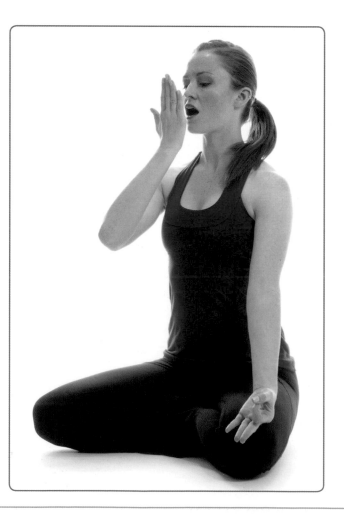

THREE-PART BREATHING (DIRGA PRANAYAMA)

Three-part breathing is a great technique to perform at the beginning or end of your yoga practice. To prepare, sit in a comfortable cross-legged position, or lie on your back. Tune in to the natural rise and fall of your breath. If your mind is really active, notice that, too, and then just bring your attention back to the breath. Then, carry out the following steps.

1 Exhale all the air out of your body so you feel like an empty balloon. Then inhale through the nose, filling your belly with breath. You may even want to bring a hand to rest on your belly to feel this. Exhale out the nose, emptying your belly. Thinking just of the belly, inhale and exhale through your nose for several counts of 5.

2 On an inhale, bring breath into your belly and then into your rib cage. Imagine your belly filling with air and then extra air rising into the rib cage, slightly parting the ribs. Exhale through your nose, emptying your rib cage and then your belly. On your exhale you can imagine your navel pulling in gently toward your spine. Repeat for a few more breaths.

3 On an inhalation, breath into your belly, then your rib cage, then your upper chest. Feel your heart-center light up with breath, filling and rising. Exhaling, release the air from your heart-center, then rib cage, then belly. Inhale and exhale through the nose several times like this, imagining the air touching all three parts of your body: belly, lungs/rib cage, and heart/chest. Exhaling, imagine the breath leaving each area. Perform about ten breaths.

YOGIC INSPIRATION

Beyond igniting your body with energy, yoga can inspire the imagination. The word *inspire* comes from Latin roots meaning "to breathe life into." With the continuous breathing, moving, and concentrating it demands, yoga can really ignite the imagination.

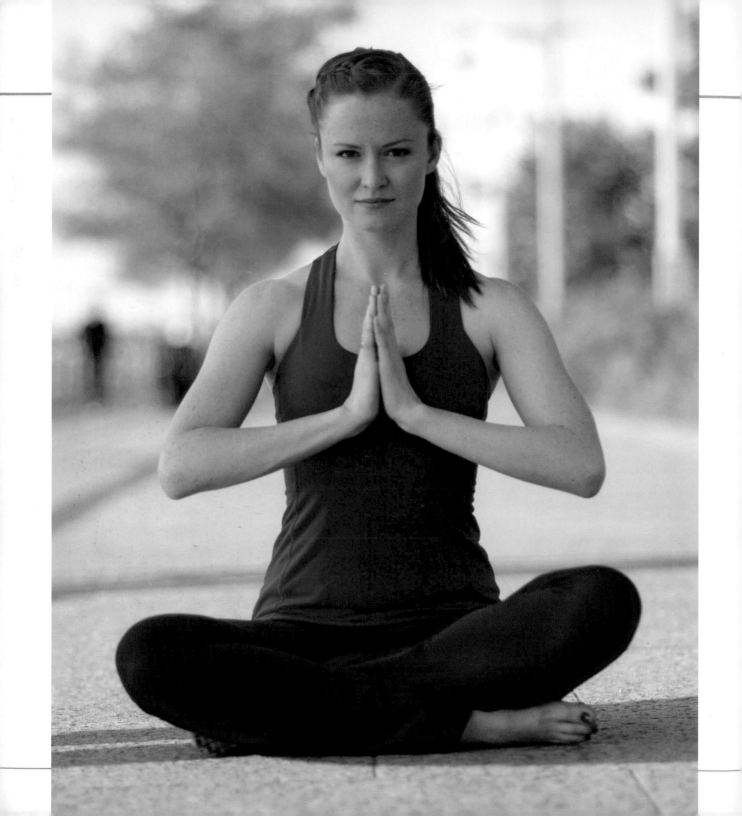

ALTERNATE-NOSTRIL BREATHING

Alternate-nostril breathing may feel strange at first, but it is a wonderfully effective technique for balancing the emotions, evening out thoughts, and bringing a sense of calm to the body. To prepare, sit up tall.

To practice alternate-nostril breathing, you will need to use a hand position to allow you to breathe through one nostril at a time. Begin and end this breath with the left side of the nose, following these steps.

1 Allow your left hand to rest in your lap and raise your right. Curl your pointer and middle fingers into the palm of your hand so only the thumb, ring finger, and pinky are extended.

2 Bring the thumb of your right hand to rest just above your right nostril. Bring your ring finger to rest just above your left nostril.

3 Press your thumb into your right nostril, closing it off. Exhale through your left nostril only. Then, inhale through your left nostril.

4 Close off both nostrils using your thumb and finger, and then exhale out your right nostril, allowing your thumb to lift up.

5 Inhale through your right nostril, close off both, then exhale through your left.

6 It can be helpful to add a count to this breath. For instance, try inhaling, exhaling, and hold for a count of 4.

7 After a few rounds, exhale out your left nostril and allow your right hand to rest in your lap. Sit for a few minutes after practicing and allow your breath to return to normal. See if you notice any difference between how you feel after the breathing versus before.

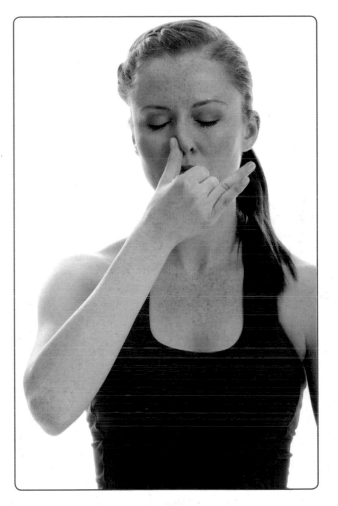

BREATH OF FIRE (BHASTRIKA PRANAYAMA)

Practicing the energizing breath Breath of Fire, or Bhastrika Pranayama, involves pumping the breath in and out at equal intervals, focusing on the belly and nose to stoke what feels like a fire within. For step-by-step instructions, turn to page 91.

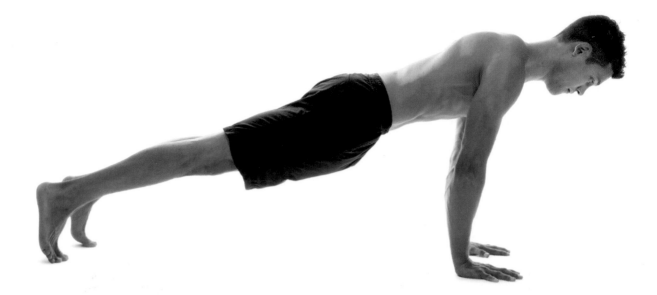

TRANSITIONING BETWEEN POSES

First and foremost, it is the breath that guides yoga transitions. You may, for instance, move through your Sun Salutations with one breath per movement, inhaling as you lift your arms up into Mountain Pose, exhaling into Forward Fold, and so forth throughout your practice.

Instead of rushing from one pose to the next, try to explore the space in between poses. Allow yourself to feel all the steps of the transition. In yoga, we are constantly moving, but can achieve quite a stillness inside during even the most fast-moving sequence. Conversely, when we are sitting still in yoga we are actually still moving in that the breath never stops, and we are paying close attention to what is going on within our bodies, even when sitting motionless with eyes closed.

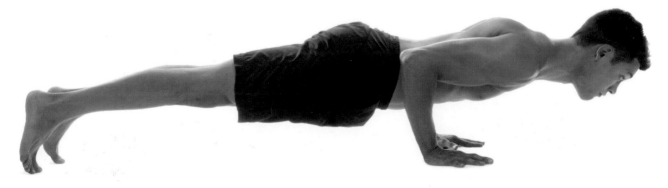

COUNTER POSE

To keep a joint as healthy as possible, it is beneficial to move it in multiple ways. If you bend forward, you should counter that pose by then performing a backbend to balance out the movement. Performing counter poses also help to balance out energy within the body.

You hear a lot about "letting go" in yoga. Yoga is really a great, practical way to practice the art of letting go. After all, you may spend much time getting into a pose and finding the shape, only to find it is now time to transition out of it and into a new shape. Just when you feel you have assumed the perfect Downward-Facing Dog, for example, it might be time to roll out into Plank. As often happens in life, as soon as we get something "down" the next challenge opens up. We are always learning and growing and moving. In yoga, at least, we get to practice this change with ease and grace.

So without any great pressure, challenge yourself to notice how to get into shapes and how to leave them. Notice everything that is happening in the split-seconds between movements.

GETTING MOTIVATED

Remember that the first word of the first *Yoga Sutra* is atha, translating to "now." In full, the *sutra* reads: Atha Yoga Anusasanam, or "Now the instruction of Yoga is being made. This *sutra* reminds us, in a few words, that now is the time for yoga. Yoga is not something to merely read about or study, but something to try in the here and now. Yoga is not words alone, but practice, and there is no better time to begin than right now.

Momentum is important; the more you do yoga, most likely the more you will want to keep doing it. If you have not been exercising or moving much lately, it may initially take more discipline to make your way to the yoga mat. But over time, it will become natural to you.

There are benefits to yoga beyond flexibility, strength, a calm mind, and connection to spirit. Many people feel yoga helps them to look younger and healthier. I've seen friends walk into yoga class looking very tired from the day, and leave glowing. Yoga can keep people looking youthful through good circulation, deep breathing, honest sweat, and de-stressing. Yoga can energize when you feel rundown and calm when you are frazzled.

Many also feel that yoga strengthens intuition. This makes sense; in yoga, we practice listening deeply to the body and the mind. On the physical level, you listen to your body in poses and see what feels best to you today. This constant "deep listening" practice can

translate to life off the mat and help you hear your own intuition when faced with decisions, for example.

Through tuning in to your body and treating it well through your yoga practice, you are likely to find yourself compelled to eat a more healthful diet. You may find that you want to eat more vegetables, or crave a particular protein. In this way, eating healthily becomes something that originates from the inside out, rather than a test of willpower.

THE 14TH *YOGA SUTRA*

The 14th *Yoga Sutra*, as we know, translates to: "Practice becomes firmly grounded when well attended to for a long time, without break and in all earnestness." This reminds us that practice makes practice! Not perfect. And the more we practice, the more we plant seeds for wellness in body and mind. And the more we practice with earnestness—not necessarily with seriousness, but with an authentic desire to try—the more we will benefit.

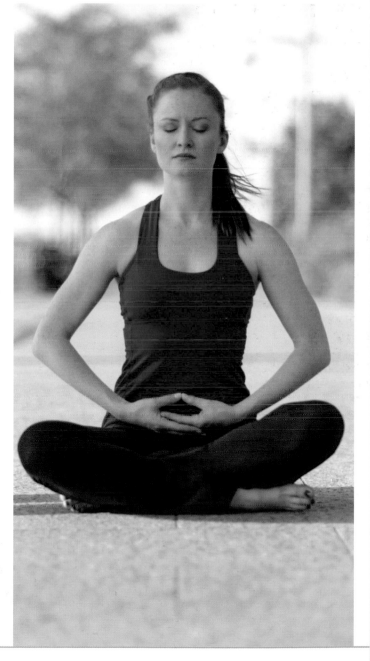

FIRING UP, NOT BURNING OUT

Yoga is about finding a balance between effort and ease. While yoga does make you feel very relaxed, often it takes some effort to get to that relaxation. It also takes discipline. However, if you push too hard you may injure yourself or forget all about the "ease" part of yoga. Nothing should hurt in yoga practice. But you should test yourself and the edges of your comfort zone.

In yoga we often talk about your "edge." Part of the practice is finding it! You have to be honest with yourself in yoga: where can you push a little further? Can you really hold the pose longer or stretch slightly more? It is vital to listen to your body. If something starts to feel painful or like you're going too far, stop. It is an advanced yoga practice to know when to back off and when to go further. You want to fire yourself up with yoga, but not burn out!

And remember, yoga is a practice. It is better to light the flame of practice every day and keep it going than to go "yoga crazy" and then fizzle or burn out on it. A little at a time can take you far.

REGULAR PRACTICE

The more often you practice yoga, the more you feel results. I didn't fully understand the benefits of yoga until I began practicing it regularly. Though I felt pretty good after one random class every once in a while, once I started practicing regularly I began to see real changes in my body, mind, and spirit. I grew stronger and more flexible all around. My mind grew more clear and calm with deeper focus.

IN BALANCE

Most of us have a fear response when faced with that moment when we might fall (and even the most accomplished yogis fall over from time to time). Balancing yoga poses are a great way to test your limits and develop bravery along with strong and supple muscles. After all, if you fall here, the mat and floor are there to catch you. The feeling of reaching beyond your comfort zone will benefit you off of the mat, too. For a Facing Fear sequence, see page 153.

My spirit was uplifted and I grew to know myself more inside. It was by regularly visiting my yoga practice that these things began to emerge.

Your daily practice may be an hour or 90 minutes, but 10 minutes a day will also yield palpable results when practiced regularly. You may only have time for a short series of poses, a sitting meditation practice, or a few poses linked with conscious breathing. Remaining fully "present" while carrying out just one or two poses may prove to be more beneficial than practicing many poses but being mentally checked out. Give yourself time to really breathe in poses, tuning in to how your body feels and what you are thinking about. Then, when you practice the next day, see if your body and mind are in the same place or a different place. By practicing yoga regularly, you will learn a lot about yourself.

SURPASSING LIMITS

Through practicing yoga with regularity, you will grow to understand what you're comfortable with, the nature of your habits, and the things that feel uncomfortable or even scary. Once you step out of your comfort zone, you will experience a palpable sense of growth. Whether you amble slowly out of this comfort zone into uncharted territory or leap into something new, you will learn something about yourself. What's important is that you dare to try:

hold that Side Plank a few breaths longer than you think you can, and launch into Crow pose even if it makes your heart skip a beat.

Remember that nothing should ever hurt in yoga, though you may feel a stretch or the shaking of new muscles being formed. To avoid strain and injury, some alignment cues—think keeping your knee aligned over your ankle in the Warrior lunges, or keeping your neck in neutral during Shoulder Stand—are important.

Know your edge. As you try the poses in this book, you may notice that some feel more "natural" and effortless than others. Notice where your body or mind gives you some resistance, and see if you can go further. Sometimes your mind may tell you that something is boring; can you try anyway? Maybe your mind will tell you, "This is too hard;" push through regardless. Maybe you'll be more inclined to practice forward folds than to do backbends; can you try it the other way around, just for fun? Yoga is essentially a playground for you to test—and try to excel—your own limits. And if we you can begin to do this on the yoga mat, we can also begin to do it in life.

QUICK FIRE-UP

It's easy to assume you should have energy before approaching your yoga mat. Many times we want to feel "up to exercising" before we roll the mat out. However, yoga itself can energize you even on the most sluggish of days. Don't let being tired, drained or fatigued stop you from practice. You may discover that yoga is a magical energizer!

For a quick pick-me-up, sit in Full Lotus pose (page 120) and practice Breath of Fire (page 91). It's like a natural shot of espresso. Try three rounds.

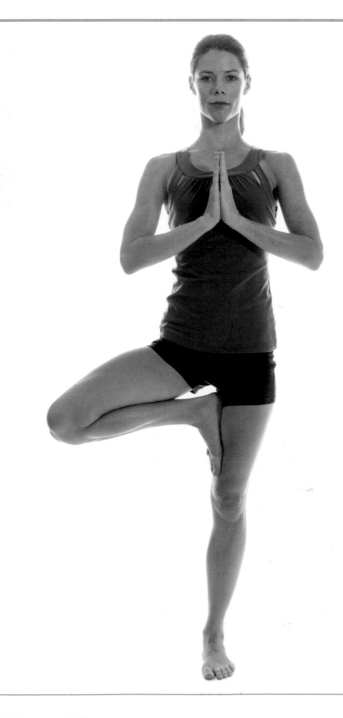

HOW TO ACE THIS COURSE

Now that you have laid the groundwork for your yoga practice, it is time to move on to the poses. The following pages provide all the information you will need to ace this course, regardless of your level of experience.

Acing this course does not mean attaining the perfect Warrior II, but rather showing up to your mat, being openminded, and really trying the Warrior II. Yoga teacher Pattabhi Jois once proclaimed, "Yoga is "99 percent practice and 1 percent theory." Another yoga teacher, Sharon Gannon, says,"Through repetition the magic arises." I thoroughly agree with them, and often tell my yoga students, "Yoga is a practice, not a perfect."

It's true: yoga is about the journey. If you keep practicing yoga, even if it's just a few minutes a few times a week, then you are "acing" it. It is a challenge in this day and age to carve out time to get to know yourself and take care of your body and mind. You are a yoga ace by making this effort.

That said, if you fall off the wagon and miss a regular practice time, that's when you get to practice other yoga lessons: forgiveness and try-try-again. There will be times in your individual yoga practice when you will fall, too. You might lose your balance during Tree Pose or stumble when transitioning from one pose to another, and that is all right. Whether you fall over in a pose or skip a day of practice, what's most important is your effort to re-engage. After all, falling over is part of life; it's what you

ROOT DOWN TO RISE UP

For standing poses, the mantra "root down to rise up" is helpful. Your foundation is vital: take a few moments to set up a strong base before you begin. You can root down into the earth in Warrior poses for example, and then feel expansion as you find your balance and reach outward.

do after the fall that matters. If you notice that you're beating yourself up after taking a fall, practice doing the opposite—and then try again.

Instructions in this book will be provided in a step-by-step way. I encourage you to be mindful of all steps and try not to just rush into a pose. Most yoga poses have many variations, versions that are simpler for beginners and more advanced for experienced practitioners. Accordingly, you will find variations listed alongside many of the yoga poses in the following pages.

Even if a given variation is listed as "harder" than another, this does not make it "better". For instance, the goal of Forward Fold is not necessarily to touch your toes. Being able to touch your toes probably won't make you happier, or a better person....nor will it make your waistline noticeably smaller. But if you can do the modification that is right for you, with awareness, you will learn from the pose.

Once you get a pose down, in fact, it can be nice to practice it with your eyes closed. This way, yoga poses become more about a series of sensations, felt from the inside out, and less about forming a shape in space. You should be aware of the shape you are assuming, but it is also fruitful to notice whatever variation you are in and tune your senses to all the sensations there.

Pain is your body's way of saying you should try a gentler variation. And just because you are able to carry out a "harder" variation on

BE GENTLE

Your body can change quite a bit, so don't be discouraged if you do not achieve "perfect" form right away. If you can't do a pose now but keep practicing, you soon will build up strength and endurance. It's wise to know when to rest.

Monday doesn't mean you will necessarily find it a breeze on Tuesday. Every time you come to the yoga mat, your body will feel different.

All of the following poses contain elements of both structure and softness. You want to challenge yourself, but you do not want to strain yourself. You should feel some muscles working and others relaxing or stretching in a pose. You should notice focus in your mind, but also a sense of ease. Yoga, in other words, is not about going totally soft and lax or being totally rigid and forceful. It's about balance.

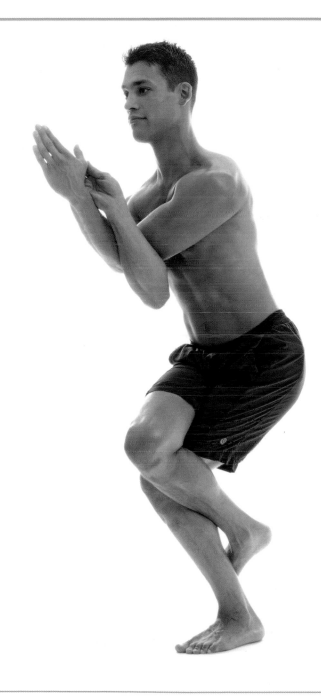

You may find that with regular practice the rest of your life off the mat takes on a different tone. It makes sense: if you're spending time getting flexible, strong and calm, you will approach your daily activities with strength, ease, and steadiness. Along the way, this regular practice will make your body leaner and stronger. You may even find yourself sleeping better along with eating more healthily.

The yoga poses in your Essential Course work with the natural movements of your body. For example, instead of pushing through sets of squats for strong legs, you may hold a few rounds of Thunderbolt Twist, deeply breathing and checking out what is going on inside. Your body responds to this and naturally becomes stronger and more relaxed. And when your body feels this way, changes often begin to occur from the inside out.

Yoga can be dipped into throughout the day—before work, as a mid-day pick-me-up, or before bed as a soother. I have a friend who regularly shuts her Manhattan office door around four o'clock, when she gets that late-afternoon energy slump, to stand on her head. Going upside down gives her energy, and is longer lasting and healthier than eating a candy bar for a burst. Many people love to do some restorative poses before bed, to settle both an active mind and calm the body. Yoga gives us tools we can use all day long.

BE AWARE OF BREATH

As you're holding the poses, try to notice the quality of your breath. See if you can keep it long, and work with ujjayi breath (see page 23). If the breath ever becomes choppy or held, you may be straining—in which case you should come into Child's Pose (page 132) and take a few breaths to relax and reconnect to the present moment.

II. YOUR ESSENTIAL COURSE

Your Essential Course consists of six lessons, each with eight exercises. Complete with minute-by-minute instructions, each lesson is designed to last one hour. Repetition is vital to learning yoga, and if you devote time to learning these poses they should eventually become second nature. The course allows time to explore each pose, feeling which parts of it come easily and which are more challenging. By taking just one hour to explore these poses step by step, you will end up with a toolkit of yoga poses which you can use —and build upon —as your yoga practice evolves.

Essential Yoga does not need to be taken all at once. Rather, the following lessons are designed for busy people. You may be squeezing your yoga sessions into various times during morning, noon, or evening —and accordingly, though they can be practiced any time, these 6 lessons are designed to mirror the energetic arc of a day. There are poses for the morning, when you may feel sluggish but are preparing for a long series of activities ahead of you; for mid-day, when your energy might be bright and high like the sun; and for the end of the day, when you are settling in and winding down.

You will begin by learning the elements of the Sun Salutations, which are themselves invigorating when practiced first thing in the morning. Then you'll embark on some balancing poses, which may be appropriate to learn and practice during the late morning, when your focus is sharp and your body is open to the challenges of standing on one leg in Dancer's Pose, take flight into Side Crow, and more. Next, you'll explore poses that work your core muscles, strengthening the powerhouse from which all bodily movement originates and giving you a leaner, tighter midsection in the process.

EXTRA CREDIT
Let your breath guide you. In general, when we reach up and out and extend, we inhale. When we compress, fold forward, and move within, we exhale.

Moving into the second half of your Essential Course, you will burn calories through the challenging Fire Up poses, which may come in handy to counteract afternoon slump. Then, it will be time to twist yourself every which way like a pretzel, getting fitter and fitter until you are finally ready to meditate in Full Lotus Pose. Finally, you will learn a series of poses that will help you wind down before bed.

At the end of the book, you will apply your knowledge in a series of yoga flows, all designed to give you maximum benefit even if you have minimal time to spare.

SALUTE THE SUN

In the following lesson, you will learn how to carry out the poses that form the basis for yoga's Sun Salutations—those flowing postures, linked by breath, that are usually practiced at the beginning of a yoga practice, warming the body much like the sun warms up the earth. As you inhale and exhale your way through these poses, you will awaken your body and mind. Focus on both shaking off lethargy and letting go of extra scattered energy as you cultivate a feeling of centeredness.

After carrying out your one-hour lesson, turn to pages 142–143 to put these poses together in Sun Salutations A and B. Through the Sun Salutations, you create heat within your body. This can help with stretching later in the practice, or simply get you warmed up for what lies ahead. When you shift position with regularity, your body moves like a metronome, which can be very soothing and invigorating at the same time—giving you a shot of focus to draw upon all day long.

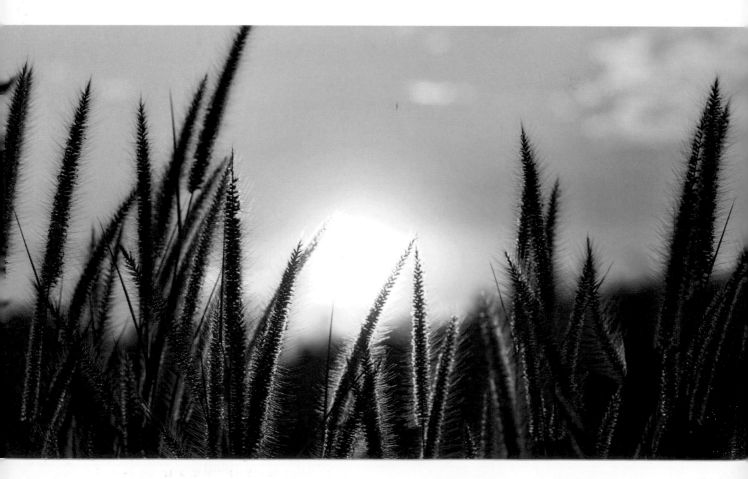

MOUNTAIN POSE | TADASASANA

Mountain Pose will give you stability and strength, a feeling of openheartedness, and the sense of clarity that comes from simply looking straight ahead. The alignment points found in Mountain Pose form the basis of many other standing poses. Let the openness of the front of your body remind you to be receptive, and the strength of the back of your body remind you that you can hold yourself up in confidence.

1 Stand with your toes and heels touching. Allow your feet to root into the floor, your body weight distributed evenly through all four corners of each foot: the big toe, little toe, inner heel, and outer heel.

2 Slightly tuck your tailbone, pulling your belly button toward your spine. Gently engage your core. Make sure your chin is parallel to the floor.

3 On an inhalation, raise your shoulders; exhaling, lower them, pressing back and away from your ears. Broaden your chest. Keep your face soft, your chin parallel to the floor. Hold.

Spend **2 minutes** holding the pose, concentrating on your standing alignment. Cultivate a sense of focus for what lies ahead.

While you stand in Mountain Pose, practice Three Part Breathing. Breathe into your belly, your chest, and finally your throat. Then, breathe out from your throat, then your chest, and finally your belly.

EXTRA CREDIT As you begin the pose, try rocking forward and backward and then side to side to find strong, even ground. Here, you "root down to rise up"; with a strong connection to the earth, any pose can more readily grow. Imagine a thin thread attached the crown of your head, lightly tugging you upward.

FORWARD FOLD | UTTANASANA

Practicing Forward Fold is a reminder to let your head fall below the heart for a while. On stressful days when your mind is busy, you can use take a moment to perform Forward Fold as you imagine worried thoughts pouring from the top of your head into the floor. Allow yourself to let go and as your heart symbolically leads the way.

The following steps describe a deep fold, with hands grasping ankles, but Forward Fold can also be a more gentle stretch; see Variations for some ideas. Above all, this pose is about release.

1 From Mountain Pose, inhale and bring your arms overhead.

2 Exhale, hinge forward from your hips and begin to fold your upper body forward. Move slowly and with control. At the point where your fingertips reach the floor, flatten your back. This is Half Lift.

3 Let your upper body "fall" over your legs. Reaching your fingers to the floor and then, if you feel comfortable, deepen your stretch by grasping your ankles. Draw your upper body closer and closer to your legs as you hold.

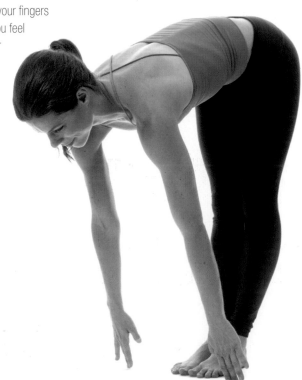

Take **2 minutes** to find the pose and hold it. Then rise up to Mountain Pose.

Spend **5 minutes** going back and forth between Mountain Pose and Forward Fold. Try each of the three easier variations of Forward Fold to add variety. Notice which variation feels most natural to you. This sequence is sometimes referred to as Wave.

On your last Mountain Pose, take a big inhale and reach your arms overhead. Arch backward and hold. Imagine your heart opening.

Release into Forward Fold, and then rise into Half Lift in preparation for Plank.

VARIATIONS

Easier
For a slightly easier stretch, hold the pose with your hands resting on the floor instead of grasping your ankles. Your fingers can point either toward your feet (as shown) or away from them.

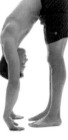

Easier
For a gentler stretch, try grasping your opposite elbows with both hands.

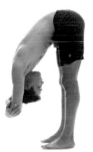

Easier
You can make the stretch easier by bending your knees softly.

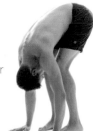

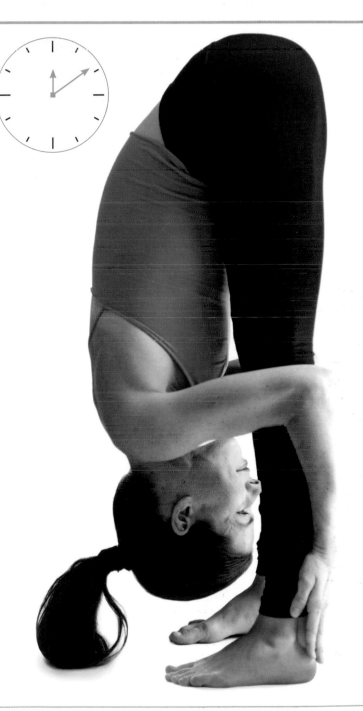

PLANK

Plank looks a lot like the extended-arm part of a push-up. In yoga, we often move into this pose from a low lunge position by stepping one foot back to meet the other, or from moving into it from Forward Fold as described below.

This pose accomplishes a lot. Engaging both upper and lower body, Plank strengthens your core and arms. While it is an important step in the Sun Salutations, where it is generally held for just one breath, it is also beneficial when practiced on its own. Start by holding for three breaths and then five, working your way up to longer and longer holds.

1 From Half Lift, bend your knees, place your hands on the floor outside of your feet, fingers spread wide. One by one, step your feet back to an upper push-up position. Your wrists and shoulders should be stacked and your toes curled under. Push through your heels and engage your legs and core. Gaze downward, pressing your shoulders back and down to avoid tensing your neck.

2 Hold, breathing comfortably. Visualize your body forming a straight line of energy, from the crown through your spine and down to your heels. Press away from the floor lightly.

Spend **5 minutes** practicing Plank, starting with the easier variation if desired. Come in and out of the shape, aiming to hold the position as long as possible while maintain your alignment and breathing deeply. You'll feel heat building in your body.

As you reach the end of your last hold, instead of releasing, remain in Plank in preparation for Chaturanga.

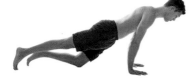

Easier
One by one, bring your knees to the floor and keep them there as you hold Plank. Through practicing this variation over time, you will build upper body and core strength to extend your legs into the full expression of the pose.

EXTRA CREDIT For a strong foundation, ensure that your wrists and shoulders are stacked. Your hands should be planted shoulder-width apart with palms pressed flat and fingers spread wide. Your hips should be in line with the shoulders. To help with this—and derive optimal ab-toning benefit—think of engaging your belly so there's no sway in your lower back.

CHATURANGA | CHATURANGA DANDASANA

Chaturanga is a pose we exhale through as we transition from one pose to the next—usually from Plank to Upward-Facing Dog—during a Sun Salutation. You can think of it as a point where you shift from the upper to the lower positions of a push-up.

However, performed on its own, Chaturanga actually gives you an intense strengthening workout. As you lower into Chaturanga and then hold it, your abs must stay engaged as yor arms work very hard to maintain your body's straight line. Let your breath (and willpower) guide you through these holds as you push firmly downward through your heels.

1 From an upper push-up position, or Plank, inhale to prepare.

2 Exhale and slowly begin lowering your body to the floor, bending your arms.

3 Engage your core muscles. Keep your elbows close to your body, pointing them back as you continue to bend and lower.

4 Once you are halfway to the floor, stop and hold.

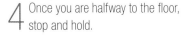

Spend **5 minutes** exploring the pose, starting with the easier variation if desired. Hold each repetition for as long as possible.

Now for a potent arm and abdominal challenge: For **3 full minutes,** practice the transition between Plank and Chaturanga, starting with the easier variations before working up to the full expressions of both poses. Your elbows should be pointed upward, not outward, throughout this yogic push-up.

Hold your last Chaturanga in preparation for Upward-Facing Dog.

VARIATIONS

Easier
Chaturanga takes a lot of upper body strength. As you are developing this strength, place your knees on the floor and keep them grounded there as you move from Plank to Chaturanga and hold.

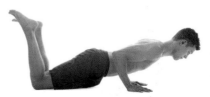

EXTRA CREDIT This Sun Salutation staple is a powerful abdominal toner. You may feel your abs shaking as you adopt this position. Challenge yourself to breathe through any discomfort that you may feel as you work toward a more streamlined midsection.

UPWARD-FACING DOG | URDHVA MUKHA SVANASANA

Upward-Facing Dog is an important part of the Sun Salutations, where it is usually held for one to three breaths. When practiced on its own, it is beneficial for opening up the front of your body—your throat, shoulders, and chest (including, symbolically, your heart). It also stretches your spine, and is a potent toner for the abdominal muscles. Assuming Upward-Facing Dog is a great, energizing way to start the day.

1 Lie facedown on the floor. Assume a lower push-up position. Your arms should be bent so that they form right angles, with your upper arms in line with your torso. Press into the floor with your hands, fingers facing forward.

2 Position your feet so that you are balancing on your toes, heels to the ceiling. Your entire body should form a straight line, with your legs fully extended. Your back and neck should be in a neutral position. Gaze toward the floor.

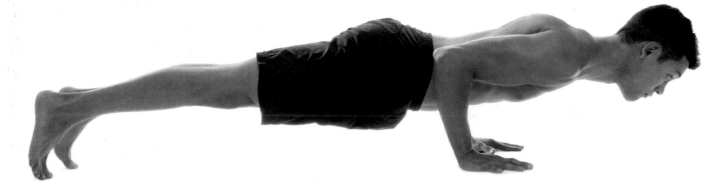

Give yourself **5 minutes** to explore this pose. Hold, release, and then assume Chaturanga to begin again. Now, you're ready to run through the sequence from the beginning. In **2 minutes,** carry out Mountain Pose, Forward Fold, Plank, Chaturanga, and then Upward-Facing Dog, holding each for two to three breaths. You should feel your body and mind revving up!

EXTRA CREDIT To hold the pose longer and stronger, activate your fingertips rather than pressing down your palms. Your fingers should be widely spread, your hands positioned directly underneath your shoulders.

3 On an inhalation, arch your back and press your palms into the floor. At the same time, lift your upper chest. As you perform this movement, pull your abdominal muscles inward, imagining your navel being drawn back toward your spine.

4 Balance so that your knees are positioned a few inches off your floor. Draw strength from your core muscles; it should be your strongly engaged abdominal muscles, not your toes, that provide support and stability as you perform the pose. Activate through your arms, continuing to press down into the floor with your hands.

5 Roll your shoulders back and down, pressing them away from your ears. On an inhalation, arch your back more deeply and allow the arch to extend through your neck. Tilt your head back, lifting your gaze toward the ceiling.

6 Hold for three full breaths, building up to longer if desired.

EXTRA CREDIT For a wonderfully invigorating stretching session, practice flowing from Upward-Facing Dog to Downward-Facing Dog and then back again. Let your breath guide you. Inhale to stretch forward and bend back into Upward-Facing dog, and then exhale as you curl your toes under, lift your hips, and press down into your heels to move into Upward-Facing Dog.

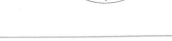

DOWNWARD-FACING DOG | ADHO MUKHA SVANASANA

Downward-Facing Dog is an important foundation pose and integral to the Sun Salutations. If you practice it on its own in the morning, you'll reap benefits too. A great way to cultivate strength and build flexibility, this pose is highly energizing. As you hold your body in an upside-down V shape, imagine that you have a line of energy shooting from the top of your head up your spine and out your sit bones. Imagine you have another line of energy shooting down your legs, tailbone to heels. As in Forward Fold, your heart presides above your head in Downward-Facing Dog. As you hold this inverted posture, imagine changing your orientation to the world.

1 Kneel on your hands and knees, with your fingers pointed forward. Curl your toes under, and inhale to prepare.

2 Exhale, and press your hands down into the floor as you lift your tail bone toward the ceiling, straightening your legs until your body takes on the shape of an upside-down V. Your hands should stay anchored to the floor, and your feet should now be flat against the floor.

3 Take a moment to perfect your form. Spread your fingers wide and ensure your wrists are parallel to the front of the mat. Your arms and hands should stay actively engaged. Reach your heels toward the floor. Engage your core, pulling your navel inward. Hold.

EXTRA CREDIT As you hold, focus on your legs. Try to straighten your knees, press your heels into the floor, and turn your thighs very slightly inward. With your hands, press down into the floor.

Take **5 minutes** to assume, hold, and then repeat the pose, paying attention to your form.

Unfold into Plank. Move into Chaturanga and then Upward-Facing Dog. Press your palms into the floor and move into Downward-Facing Dog. Spend **3 minutes** carrying out this sequence several times until the transitions feel natural, spurred by your breath.

Take **2 minutes** to run through the entire sequence, beginning with Mountain Pose. When you reach Downward-Facing Dog, hold the pose in preparation for Warrior I.

DOWNWARD-FACING DOG | Adho Mukha Svanasana

WARRIOR I | VIRABHADRASANA I

When you assume Warrior I, you will feel strong and energized. Take time at the beginning to adjust your feet; a strong foundation is important. Feel your connection to the ground through your feet before you reach toward the sky with your arms and your chest. Feel free to shorten or widen your stance; the important thing is to have a strong foundation from which to reach out. Keep your hips square and facing forward. If you had headlights on your hips they would be shining straight forward, lighting up the room. When performed as part of the Sun Salutations, we may move through this shape in one breath, with one movement.

1 From Downward-Facing dog, inhale and lift your left leg upward.

2 Exhale and draw the foot through, placing it between your hands. Release your right heel down to the floor. Take a moment to line up the toes with the fingertips.

3 Inhale your arms overhead. Think of squaring your hips and shoulders to the front of the room. Relax your shoulders away from your ears and keep your arms active and straight.

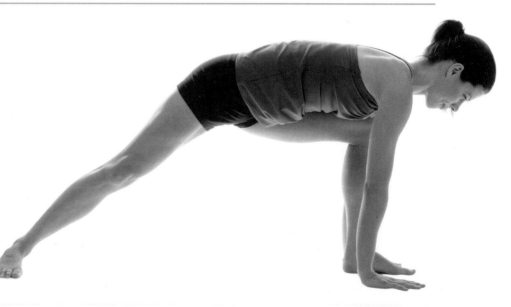

Allow yourself **6 minutes** to adopt and grow comfortable with Warrior I. Make sure to perform the pose on both sides.

In **4 minutes,** run through the whole sequence twice, ending the first sequence with Warrior I on the right side and ending the second with Warrior I on the left. Enjoy the feeling of power that will surely be coursing through your veins!

4 Exhale to deepen into the lunge, keeping your front knee stacked over the ankle.

5 Inhale and reach forward. Raise your upper body so your shoulders and hips face your front foot.

EXTRA CREDIT With each exhale, sink a bit further into the pose, keeping your front knee over the ankle. With each inhale, think of reaching toward the ceiling, from the waist up. As you hold, your lower body should stay frozen in place as your upper body reaches.

6 Roll your shoulders away from the ears, keep your fingertips active, and relax your face. Hold for three to five breaths.

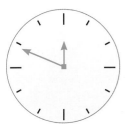

7 To transition out of the shape, exhale your hands back down, framing the foot. Repeat on the other side.

WARRIOR II | **VIRABHADRASANA II**

Warrior II is a great strengthener for your lower body. It is also an effective hip opener, which comes in handy when you've been sitting behind a steering wheel or a desk for many hours. Drawing on the fierce determination of the archetypal warrior, this pose builds focus, fortitude, and flexibility. Try holding the position a bit longer than you are initially inclined to hold it. Allow your tailbone to tuck underneath you, with the core engaged. If you had headlights on your hips, they'd be shining toward the side wall.

1 From Warrior I, inhale and look upward toward your fingertips.

2 Exhale, opening your hips as you extend your arms out to your sides to form a straight time. Gaze over your front fingertips.

3 Relax your shoulders, pressing them away from your ears. Hold the pose. With each inhale, feel yourself growing larger and taking up space; with each exhale, sink further straight downward, keeping the front knee stacked over your ankle.

EXTRA CREDIT To make sure your front knee maintains proper and safe alignment, glance down. You should be able to see a sliver of your big toe poking out from the inside of your knee.

Give yourself **6 minutes** to learn Warrior II. Carry out the pose on both sides.

Finally, run through the entire sequence twice in **5 minutes,** performing Warrior II first on the right and then on the left to complete your hourlong lesson. You are now ready to Salute the Sun every single morning.

BALANCE THAT BODY

The following lesson will challenge your sense of balance. For instance, you'll find yourself standing on one leg, and then assume daring shapes; using your toes and feet to challenge your balance and even learning to support your body weight with your arms.

Your gaze is essential to balance. As you adopt a pose and are ready to find your balance, choose one spot, or *drishti*, on which to fix your eyes as you hold. Let your gaze be soft but steady; your *drishti* should serve as your anchor, calming any frenzied thoughts, encouraging steady breath, and helping you find a sense of stability and solidity in your body.

Hold the poses as long as you can and you'll soon find your ability to focus improving exponentially. This sense of focus, combined with the perseverance and fortitude that these poses cultivate, will come in handy when other aspects of life challenge you. Notice how you feel and think when the balancing gets tough; if you notice without judgement, you may learn a lot about yourself. Notice how balancing on one side may be different from balancing on the other side, and how your balance may naturally shift from day to day. Remember that whenever you fall over, you are being given a great opportunity to get up and try again.

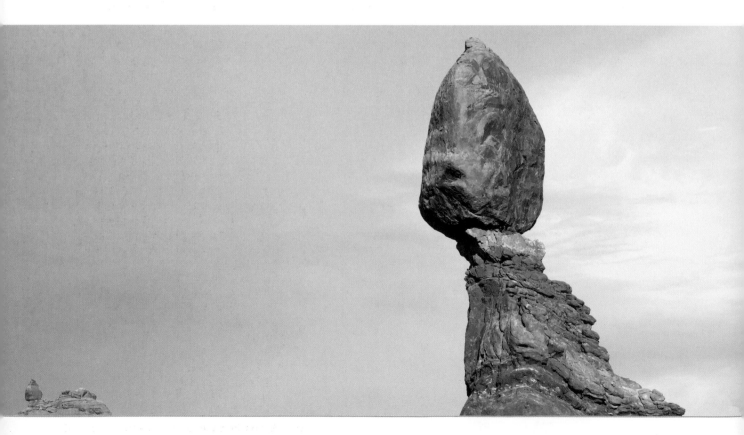

SPINAL ARM BALANCE

Spinal Arm Balance is an excellent pose for strengthening your core as well as your back. While the movement is relatively small, you are really working your abdominal muscles here as your sense of balance is challenged. Lift your arm and leg only as high as you can go while maintaining your form. If you are finding the balance difficult, feel free to leave your back leg extended on the ground at first, with toes curled under; you will still derive benefit from this position as long as you reach up and extend out.

1 Kneel on all fours. Stack your shoulders over your wrists, and your knees over your hips. Your spine should be neutral, all the way through your neck. Spread your fingers wide, your wrist creases running parallel to the front of your mat. Inhale to prepare.

2 Exhale, and extend one arm and the opposite leg simultaneously. Press firmly downward with your hand on the mat. Pull your abs inward, which will help with balance while enhancing toning benefits. Hold for three to five breaths, reaching a little further with each exhalation. Gaze upward and into the area in front of you.

3 On an exhalation, bring your arm and leg back to starting position. Repeat on the other side.

Take **1 minute** to familiarize yourself with each step of the exercise. Then, alternating, perform three slow repetitions on each side for a total of **2 minutes**. Inhale as you reach, and exhale as you bring your arm and opposite leg back to starting position. Try not to lose your balance when you switch sides. When you are balancing on one arm and one leg, try holding, motionless, for a breath or two.

Once you become comfortable with this movement, spend **2 minutes** performing faster repetitions without compromising your form or wobbling. Keep breathing, and use your core muscles to find stability.

TREE POSE | VRKSASANA

Tree Pose helps to cultivate our sense of balance. By standing on one leg, calming the breath, and finding a point of visual focus (*drishti*), we teach our minds and bodies to find balance and calm even when things feel off-center. In Tree pose, the standing foot becomes the roots, the core of the body is stable like a trunk, and the arms become like branches, able to move. Just like a tree. you may sway—but strive to stay grounded. Looking at one point of focus helps. If you do fall, just try again. Moments of falling out of poses are opportunities to see how we react to adversity in general. Because Tree Pose takes focus, it is a way to invigorate the body and mind in the morning.

1 Stand in Mountain Pose (page 43), with your hands pressed together at your heart. Shift your weight onto your left foot, feeling it steady on the floor.

2 Lift your right foot and, using your hands if desired, place it above or below your left knee. (Avoid placing the foot directly on the knee.) Try to press the foot into your left shin or thigh.

3 Hold for 5 deep breaths. Relax, letting your shoulders drop away from your ears. Keep your head upright, chin parallel to the floor.

4 Exhaling, release into Mountain Pose. Repeat on the other side.

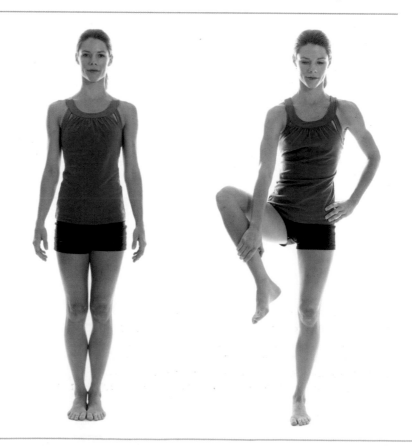

VARIATIONS

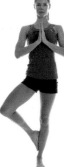

Easier
If you find the full pose uncomfortable at first, start by placing your foot below our knee.

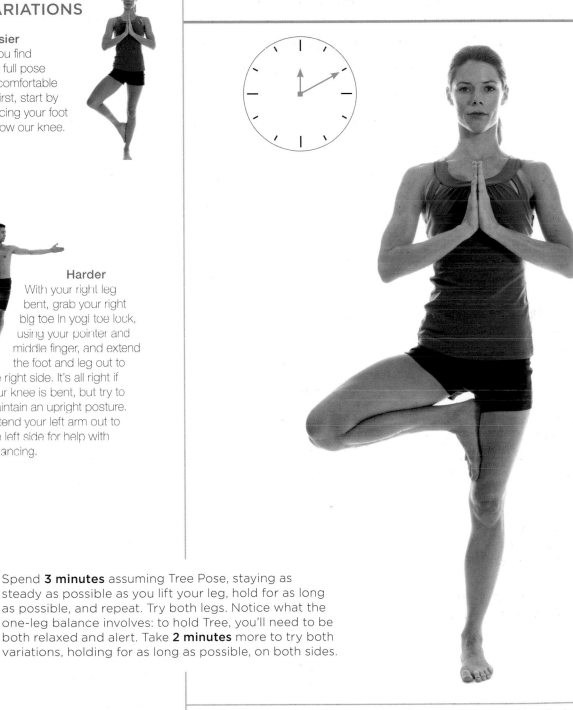

Harder
With your right leg bent, grab your right big toe in yogi toe lock, using your pointer and middle finger, and extend the foot and leg out to the right side. It's all right if your knee is bent, but try to maintain an upright posture. Extend your left arm out to the left side for help with balancing.

Spend **3 minutes** assuming Tree Pose, staying as steady as possible as you lift your leg, hold for as long as possible, and repeat. Try both legs. Notice what the one-leg balance involves: to hold Tree, you'll need to be both relaxed and alert. Take **2 minutes** more to try both variations, holding for as long as possible, on both sides.

STANDING SPLIT | URDHVA PRASARITA EKA PADASANA

Standing Split offers a phenomenal stretch for your legs, which you will feel throughout your quadriceps and hamstrings. It also brings with it all the benefits that come with going upside down, so that your head once again presides over your heart. Don't worry if you cannot lift your leg as high as you'd like. It is more important that energize the leg all the way through to your toes. Make sure you perform this challenging balance on both sides.

1 From Forward Fold (page 44), bring your weight onto your left foot.

2 Raise your right foot off the floor. Walk your fingers back in line with your toes.

3 Drop your head completely. Extend your right leg as high as possible, pointing all the way through the toes.

4 If desired, pause here for a breath or two. Once you have found your balance, deepen the stretch by grasping your left ankle with your left hand. Hold for five to eight breaths, pulling your upper body closer to your standing leg with each breath. Release, coming into Forward Fold. Repeat on the other side.

Allow yourself **3 minutes** to explore Standing Split on both sides. Embrace the new perspective that this heart-over-head position affords. Keep your hips totally square; this is more important than the height of your lifted leg. The longer you can balance, the more flexible you will become. Once you become comfortable, **1 minute** challenging your balance by lifting one arm and then the other. After practicing this pose, you should feel invigorated by the reversed blood flow.

EXTRA CREDIT

You may find that you can raise your left leg considerably higher than your right, or vice versa. That is perfectly normal, as flexibility and the ability of balance can vary from one side of your body to the other.

BIRD OF PARADISE | SVARGA DVIDASANA

Bird of Paradise is an advanced balancing pose that takes time to master. Be patient with yourself; for instance, allow yourself to bend your knees as you reach with one hand to grasp the other, and feel free to rest along the way and hold the pose at any of the challenging steps as you make your way to the full expression. Bird of Paradise offers an excellent stretch for your extended leg and hip. When you carry out the full pose, you will feel like a bird in full plumage.

1 Assume Forward Fold (page 44), with your feet hip-width apart. Weave your left arm through your legs. Begin to shift your body weight onto your right foot.

2 Inhale and then exhale, pressing into your right foot as you gradually rise up to stand. Engage your core muscles to pull you upward. Your left leg will be bend over your hand lock. Hold here for two full breaths. This is Bird of Paradise's first balancing challenge.

3 Inhale and then exhale, extending your left leg as straight as possible while keeping your upper body upright. Keep your left toes energized, either pointed or flexed. Hold for five breaths.

4 To come out of the shape, bend your left knee. Slowly and with control, lower into Standing Forward Fold, keeping your arms wrapped around your leg. Then, release your arms and let them dangle freely. Repeat on the other side.

EXTRA CREDIT For an extra balancing challenge, turn your head toward the right while your left leg is extended (and vice versa).

This empowering pose takes a while to get right. Allow yourself **7 minutes** to explore it step by step. Pause and breathe between steps whenever desired. Perform on both legs, holding for as long as possible before releasing and repeating.

WARRIOR III | **VIRABHADRASANA III**

Warrior III is an adventurous balance that strengthens your legs and ankles as well as the muscles of the back. It improves balance and will give you a sense of empowerment. To help with balancing, keep your gaze in front of the standing foot, soft and steady. Try flexing through your back foot.

1 Stand in Warrior I pose (page 54). Gaze to the floor in front of you, about 3 feet away from your toes.

2 Take a big breath in, then exhale, tipping forward on the right foot only, slowly raising the left foot off the mat. Move your hips and shoulders parallel to the floor. Draw the navel in and use your core for support.

3 Hold for five to eight breaths. To come out of the pose, inhale and raise your arms upward as you lower your back leg to the floor.

4 Bring your feet together and stand upright. Then, repeat on the other side.

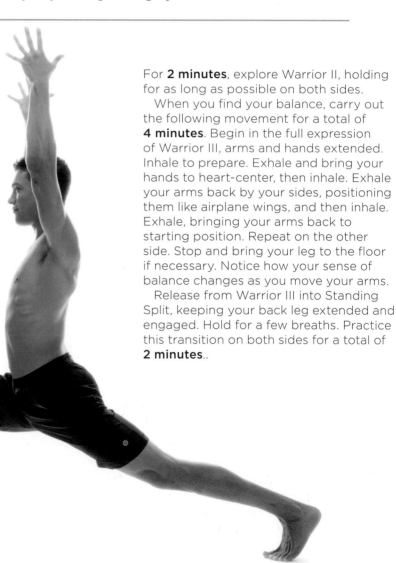

For **2 minutes**, explore Warrior II, holding for as long as possible on both sides. When you find your balance, carry out the following movement for a total of **4 minutes**. Begin in the full expression of Warrior III, arms and hands extended. Inhale to prepare. Exhale and bring your hands to heart-center, then inhale. Exhale your arms back by your sides, positioning them like airplane wings, and then inhale. Exhale, bringing your arms back to starting position. Repeat on the other side. Stop and bring your leg to the floor if necessary. Notice how your sense of balance changes as you move your arms. Release from Warrior III into Standing Split, keeping your back leg extended and engaged. Hold for a few breaths. Practice this transition on both sides for a total of **2 minutes**..

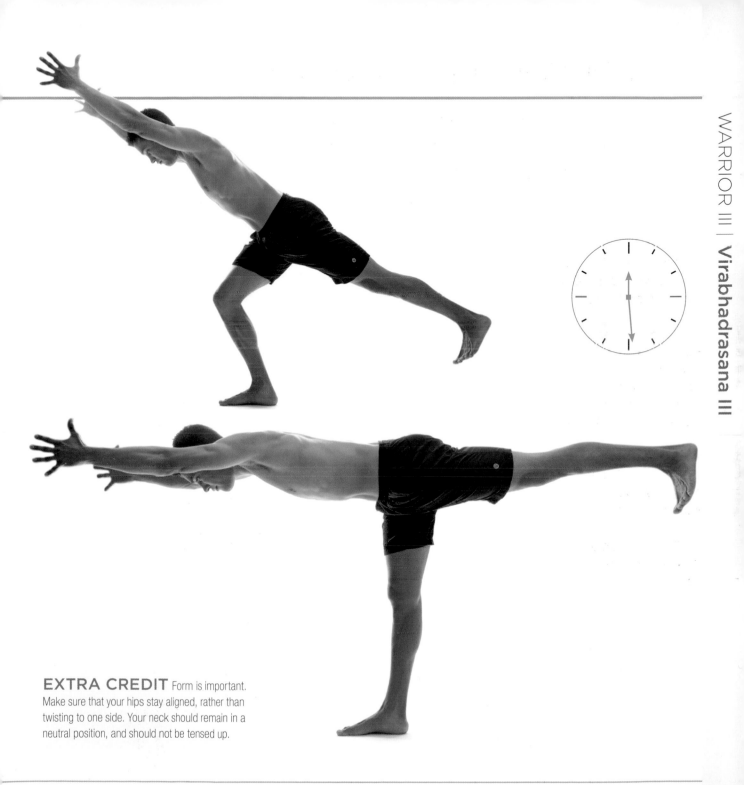

EXTRA CREDIT Form is important. Make sure that your hips stay aligned, rather than twisting to one side. Your neck should remain in a neutral position, and should not be tensed up.

DANCER'S POSE | NATARAJASANA

Considered by some to be one of the most beautiful-looking yoga poses, Dancer's Pose is an energizing balance. As you hold, gaze outward and slightly up as your chin stays parallel with the earth. Aim to keep your hips level, which can be a challenge as normally the hip of the raised leg wants to open outward. By kicking into the leg and extending through the heart, you will come into the bow shape of the dancer. Kick the leg back only a little, or not at all. Simply standing on one leg and coming into dancer's grip makes for a great Dancer's Pose.

1 Begin in Mountain Pose (page 43). Bend one leg and grab the foot from the inside, using the arm on the same side, so that you are standing on one foot.

2 Raise the arm of your standing leg. Inhale to prepare.

3 Exhale, and begin to slowly tip forward. Gaze in front of you to help with balance.

4 Use your core muscles to drive the movement as you kick your back leg into your hand, raising the leg higher as you deepen and expand the shape.

5 Hold for five breaths. With each inhale, reach further outward, and with each exhale tip further forward. Release, and then repeat on the other leg.

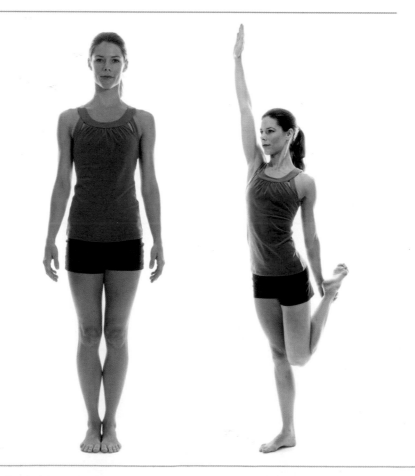

Spend **6 minutes** exploring this graceful, energizing pose. Alternating legs, balancing for as long as possible. Let your standing leg wobble, as in Tree Pose, as you reach forward and energize all the way through your fingertips as you feel both rooted and lifted.

CROW POSE | BAKASANA

Crow Pose is a fun arm balance. It can be modified to suit beginners and advanced yogis alike. If you fall, the floor isn't far, and you can come back into the shape.

1 Squat, with your feet wide apart and your hands pressed together at heart-center.

2 Bring your palms to the mat and plant them there, fingers widely spread, wrists directly below your shoulders.

3 Bend your arms and come up onto your toes. Staying here on tiptoe, rocking your weight forward and backward, is the beginning of Crow.

4 Begin to lift one toe at a time as you prepare to balance in the full posture. When you feel ready, bring the shins of your legs onto your upper arms, above your elbows.

5 Once you find your balance, gaze about 1 foot in front of you, your neck extended yet neutral. Think of leading with your heart. Hold for five breaths.

Confront this exciting pose head-on, allowing yourself **6 minutes** to explore it step by step. If you find it hard to "take flight" at first, continue trying until you balance, even if just for a few moments at first.

For **12 minutes** through the entire sequence of poses, noticing how much the sensation of balance can vary within your body. Pay attention to how poses affect you differently, both physically and emotionally. Hold Crow Pose for as long as possible at the end.

VARIATIONS

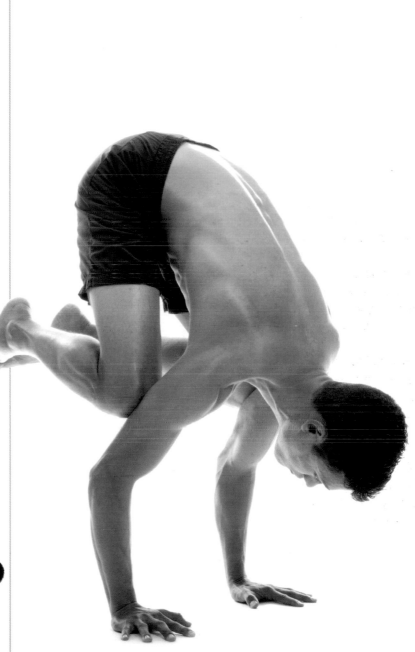

Harder

Once you grow more comfortable with Crow, bring your gaze farther in front of you, pull your belly upward, and push through the arms to achieve more height. It really does feel like flying! For advanced fun, try extending one leg or the other.

Easier

Try exploring crow pose by standing and then squatting on a block. This prop raises you up so that when you bend your elbows and bring your shins to your upper arms you will have extra room to work with. You may find it easier to tip forward into balance from a block—and when you release the pose, you can land lightly on the block.

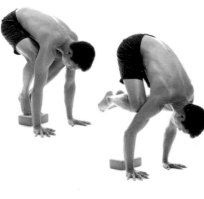

SIDE CROW POSE | PARSVA BAKASANA

Side Crow Pose is exactly what it sounds like: a Crow balance to one side. It is also an exercise in establishing a strong base before reaching outward. Before you push up, gaze at a point one foot in front of you and think of leading with your heart, as well as anchoring down into the floor with your hands.

1 Begin in a squat, then swivel your torso to the left. Place both hands flat on the mat on the outside of your left thigh. Fully extend your fingers so your hands create a firm base. The hands should stay about shoulder-width apart.

2 Bring your knees to touch. Engage your core, pulling the belly up and in; this will allow for a lighter sensation in the body, allowing you to "fly." Begin to tip your weight toward the right hands. Bring the outside edge of the right thigh to rest on the elbows of your arms. You may use both elbows, or may just use the right elbow.

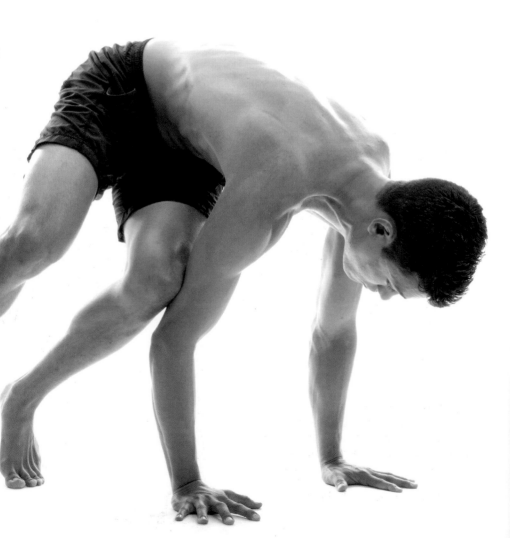

EXTRA CREDIT Attempt to connect your upper arm with the thigh to create a "shelf" for your lower body. Really engage your core, however, so you have less weight and heaviness to pick up.

3 Try lifting one foot off the floor and then the next. Push into your hands as if they were feet.

4 Hold for three to five breaths, or even longer. Focus on your breath to help you balance. Try to stay calm and breathe through any fear of falling you may feel.

5 On an exhalation, come out of the pose by softly bringing your feet to the floor. Repeat on the other side.

For **7 minutes**, take your balancing practice even further by experimenting with Side Crow. Try to find your balance on both sides, even if only for a moment. Notice how quickly your body and mind adjust to this daring balance.

YOGIC TO THE CORE

Strengthening, toning, and streamlining the core—that muscular powerhouse encompassing the back, abs, obliques, and buttocks—can immensely improve how you look and feel. In the following hour-long lesson, you will learn an array of yoga poses that do just that.

For optimal benefits, keep your core muscles engaged as you carry out these poses. You'll find that tucking your tailbone, drawing your navel in and up, and otherwise drawing upon your stomach muscles will really improve your strength and stability, helping to protect your back along the way. In fact, all yoga poses extend from the center of the body, so

the stronger this center, the more rewarding your practice! Over time, engaging your core will come to feel natural.

The following poses approach the core from different angles. Use these approaches to ignite the fire within, and then see if you can carry this core awareness with you through all of the poses in this book. In general, it is easier to feel sensations in the extremities of the body than the center. Hopefully these poses will also aid with drawing intention deeply inside and heightening sensitivity to the core of you. A sleeker, tighter, stronger midsection will be the happy byproduct.

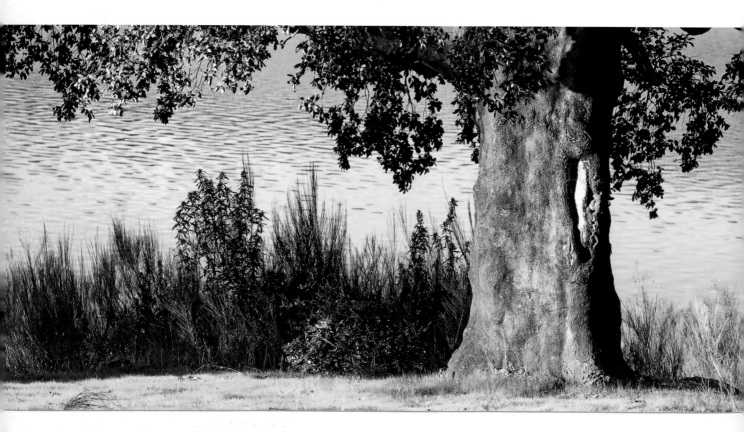

YOUR CORE BANDHAS

In yoga, a *bandha* is an inner activation that helps to direct the flow of energy within the body. Translated literally from Sanskrit, the word *bandha* means "energy lock."

Mula bandha, in turn, translates as "root lock." It involves engaging the base of the torso on the pelvic floor in order to activate the muscles at the base of the core. Sometimes tricky at first, it involves directing a deep inner muscle in and up. When you find *mula bandha*, your core naturally engages. Many advanced yogis utilize *mula bandha* during their entire practice to keep them strong, light, and invigorated as they move through poses.

You can practice *mula bandha* in conjunction with *uddiyana bandha*. To practice *uddiyana bandha*, pull your abdominal muscles inward and upward, as if they were making their way toward the area beneath your rib cage.

A good place to start: try finding both core *bandhas* in simple poses such as Mountain Pose or Downward- Facing Dog.

In Mountain Pose, imagine that your torso is a bowl holding precious liquid you don't want to spill. Tuck your tailbone to hold the imaginary bowl straight. When in this position, imagine pulling your pelvic floor up toward your navel. See if you can feel an activation that is neither too tight nor too lose.

In Downward-Facing Dog, inhale, then exhale, tucking your tailbone slightly under. Again, try to connect to the idea of your pelvic floor tucking toward your navel.

Finding core bandhas will help you to direct your energy upward, rather than losing energy, as you assume and hold yoga poses. Through engaging in the search for these core *bandhas*, you can truly lift yourself up from within as you work your core.

> Spend **4 minutes** in Mountain Pose and then Downward-Facing Dog, breathing comfortably as you find your own *mula bandha* and *uddiyana bandha*.

PLANK VARIATIONS:

SIDE PLANK

Side Plank is a powerful core strengthener. It can also impart a sense of lightness as you extend through the shape. Alignment is vital; when holding, keep your body in one long line. Do not allow your weight to sink. Instead, focus on pushing the hips up toward the ceiling to best engage your abdominal muscles, particularly the obliques.

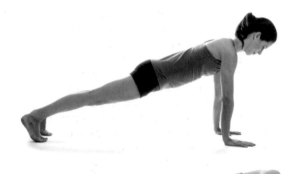

1 Begin in an upper push-up position, or Plank.

2 Bring your legs together so heels and toes touch, as if you have one strong leg instead of two.

3 Shift your weight to the left side as you roll onto the outside edge of your left foot. Try to stack your right foot and leg on top of your left. All of your weight should now rest on your left hand and the outside edge of your left foot.

4 Extend your right arm toward the ceiling. For a balance challenge, let your gaze follow the arm.

5 Keep looking at your raised arm as you hold for at least three to five breaths. Release and repeat on the other side.

Spend **3 minutes** practicing Side Plank on both sides.

FOREARM PLANK

Forearm Plank is a challenging variation of Plank. This pose quickly creates a lot of heat in the body. Try to breathe through the heat, and any resistance that you may feel as you a hold this intense core-strengthening pose. Use the breath to keep yourself going; when you feel that you cannot hold any longer, you may inhale and exhale more strongly as you hold the pose longer than you thought you could.

1 Begin in an upper push up position, or Plank, with your hands planted shoulder-width apart on the mat. Tuck your toes under.

2 Lower onto your forearms. Your body should form one straight line.

3 Push into the mat with your forearms and hold for at least five to eight breaths before releasing.

Allow yourself **2 minutes** to explore Forearm Plank, holding as long as you can while maintaining your alignment.

For **5 minutes,** carry out this powerful arm strengthener: Assume Forearm Plank. Take two full breaths. Move into Plank, placing one palm and then the other on the floor and pushing up. Step by step, move into Side Plank on the left side. Hold for two full breaths. In a smooth motion, lower your top arm and release into Plank. Move into Side Plank on the right side. Hold for two full breaths. Lower onto your forearms and hold as long as possible. Repeat if desired.

EXTRA CREDIT Avoid hunching your shoulders; instead, press them down, away from your ears.

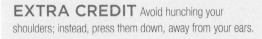

BOAT POSE | PARIPURNA NAVASANA

Boat Pose is a great way to connect with the core of your body. It strengthens your abdominals, hip flexors, spine, and thighs while also giving your hamstrings a great stretch.

1 Sit upright, with your legs extended in front of you.

2 Rock your body weight onto your sit bones. At the same time, bend your knees and lift them upward. Point your feet so that only your toes are touching the mat as you tip very slightly backward.

3 Take a moment to find your balance. Slowly and with control, extend your arms so thtat they are parallel to the floor. Keep your arms active and energized all the way through to your fingertips. If desired, hold here for a breath or two.

4 Begin to straighten your legs so that they form a 45-degree angle with the floor. Keep your chin level and your gaze forward as you hold, aiming for five breaths.

Spend **2 minutes** exploring this pose. Keep your belly pulled in throughout. While holding, take full, deep breaths. Return to step 3 and hold in preparation for Boats in Action.

EXTRA CREDIT

As you hold Boat Pose, your sense of stability should come from the powerhouse muscles of your core. Keep your core strongly engaged by breathing into your stomach.

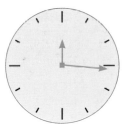

BOATS IN ACTION

Now that you have learned Boat Pose, you can put it into action. The following exercise will challenge and tone your core muscles in a dynamic way. Think of it as a yogic alternative to sit-ups. Keep your abdominal muscles pulled in and engaged throughout the movement. The better your form, the more your abdominal muscles will benefit.

1 From Boat Pose (page 78), release your extended legs to a bent position. Bring your palms together; you can think of this as your oar. Inhale to prepare.

2 Exhale, rotating toward the right, moving your arms toward the right side of your body. Look over your right shoulder. Inhale, and then exhale as you rotate back to center.

3 Repeat to the left side. Complete three rounds on both sides to give your abdominal muscles, especially your obliques, a challenging workout.

4 Return to center. Begin to release your upper body halfway toward the floor (or even lower), straightening your legs slowly as you go. This is Half Boat.

5 Hold for one full breath, then inhale, using your core muscles to pull you back up. Move slowly and with control, keeping both your arms and your legs extended.

EXTRA CREDIT Your feet may be either flexed or pointed as you carry out Boats in Action. The important thing is that your legs stay active and engaged, all the way through your toes.

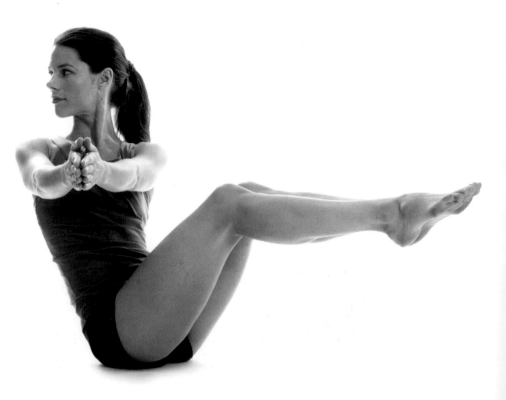

Spend **2 minutes** learning the sequence described here. Your navel should be pressed toward your spine throughout.

Devote **5 minutes** to repeating Boats in Action, going at your own pace. Let your breath guide you through this challenging, highly effective abdominal-toning sequence.

YOGA BICYCLES

Yoga Bicyles look at lot like the bicycle crunches you may remember from gym class. The difference here is the use of conscious breath: move and breathe with awareness, so you are not simply whipping through the exercise. Because this core exercise allows the back to rest on the floor, it is a very safe exercise even for yogis with sensitive backs. Remember, every time you do core work you are contributing to the overall health of your back, your spine, and the integrity of all your yoga poses across the board.

1 Lie on your back. Bring your hands behind your head, with elbows pointing out, as if you're about to do a sit-up. Bend your legs so that they form 90-degree angles, stacking knees on top of hips. Make a conscious choice to either flex or point through the feet during this exercise.

2 Inhale and draw your shoulders and upper chest up toward the knees. Use your hands only to lightly support and guide the movement, which should originate in the core.

3 Exhale, drawing your left elbow toward your left knee. Extend your left leg straight. Try not to crunch your neck.

4 On the inhale, come back to center so that your legs form 90-degree angles again.

5 Moving with your breath, inhale, then exhale, bringing the right elbow to the left knee. Continue switching sides, with one movement per breath.

Spend **2 minutes** getting familiar with every step of Yoga Bicycles. Linger in Step 2 for at least two full breaths. Press your lower body into the mat to prepare.

Launch into action: Perform ten repetitions, alternating legs. Come back to center, rest for a breath or two if desired, and then repeat. Continue for a full **6 minutes** as your obliques get strengthened and sculpted.

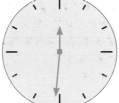

TIP TOE CAT

In yoga practice (as in life), making the smallest of adjustments can sometimes lead to profound differences. This is the case with Cat Pose. Here we will practice Tip Toe Cat by curling the toes under in traditional Cat Pose, lifting the knees just an inch or so off the mat, and using breath to activate the core. This Cat will strengthen your core from the inside out.

1 Kneel on all fours, stacking your wrists directly above your shoulders, and your knees directly over your hips. Your back and neck should be neutral, your gaze downward. Engage your abdominal muscles. Inhale to prepare.

2 Exhale and curl your tailbone under as you arch your back, pulling your navel in and up toward your spine. Allow your head to drop. This is Cat Pose.

3 Tuck your toes under and lightly lift your knees off the mat. Strongly engage your core to maintain a lift in your cat shape. Even if your knees are lifted just 1 to 3 inches off the mat, your core will have to work harder.

4 Breathe into the heat in the center of your body for three to five breaths, challenging yourself to stay perfectly still.

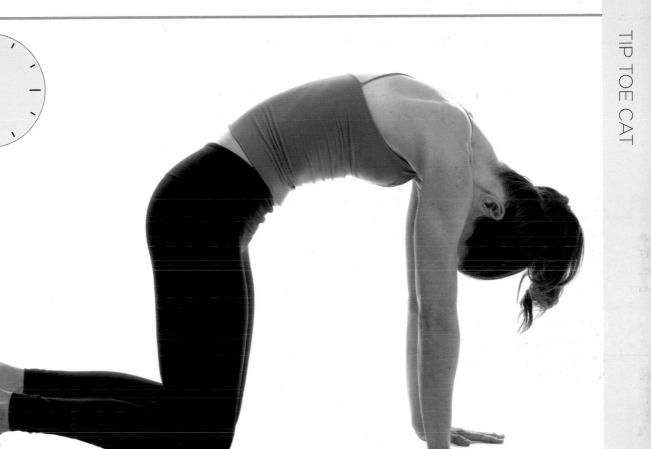

Devote **2 minutes** to finding your core *bandhas* in both the preparatory position and the arched position. Breathe deeply into your belly.

Spend **3 minutes** repeating this pose, holding for three to five breaths each time. Keep your core strongly engaged as your deep abdominal muscles grow stronger and more stable with ever breath.

EXTRA CREDIT Without your knees on the mat, your core has to work harder to maintain the pose. Lifting your knees just 1 to 3 inches will make this a highly effective abdominal strengthener.

KNEE TO NOSE

Knee to Nose is less a pose and more of a movement, or flow, one that focuses on and heats up the core. By drawing the knee to the nose, then to each elbow, you can focus on crunching and using your abdominal muscles. Use your inhales and exhales to help you move and deepen the exercise.

1 Begin in Downward Facing Dog (page 52). Inhale, and raise your right leg behind you in a straight line.

2 Exhale, beginning to draw your right knee downward and toward your chest. Engage your abdominals as you move the leg, keeping your midsection strong and stable. Press your navel toward your spine. Move slowly and with control, maintaining the upside-down V shape in the rest of your body. Try to touch knee to nose.

3 Inhale and extend your leg. Exhale and bring your knee all the way to your right elbow, so that the elbow and knee touch.

4 Inhale and extend your leg behind you. Exhale and bring your knee toward your left elbow.

5 Inhaling, lift your right leg back to extend it behind your body. Exhaling, bring the leg back to Downward-Facing dog. Hold for one breath, and then repeat on the other side.

In **2 minutes**, familiarize yourself with all steps of this pose, keeping your core engaged. Inhale as you raise your leg, and exhale as you draw it in—toward your nose, your near elbow, and then your opposite elbow. Feel a sense of "crunching" your abs as you make your belly concave.

Challenge yourself to move through the steps dynamically, without pausing, in a smooth, controlled motion. Devote **3 minutes** to one side and then **3 minutes** to the other, releasing and taking one full breath in Downward-Facing Dog once complete.

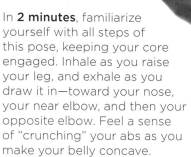

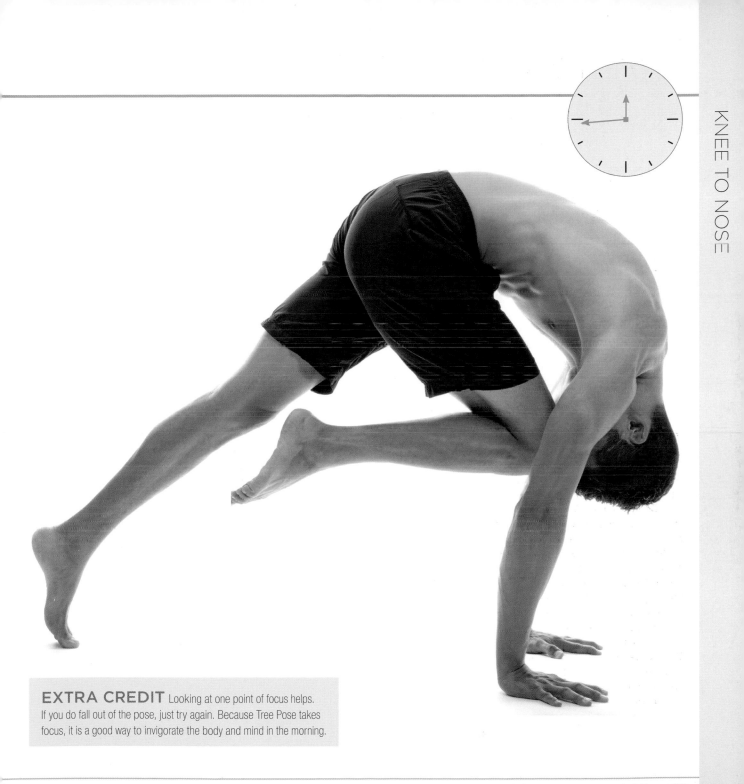

EXTRA CREDIT Looking at one point of focus helps.
If you do fall out of the pose, just try again. Because Tree Pose takes
focus, it is a good way to invigorate the body and mind in the morning.

SWING POSE | LOLASANA

When carrying out the challenging Swing Pose, you are essentially using your upper body to push the meditative Lotus position (see Full Lotus pose, page 120) into the air. This pose strengthens the upper body, but also demands a great deal of core strength for liftoff. If you find Full Lotus uncomfortable, you can still push up from "regular" crisscrossed legs—as long as you are using arm and core activation rather than just leaning on your feet. As with most yoga poses, work to keep your heart open, resisting the urge to slump your shoulders forward.

1 Sit upright in Full Lotus Pose, or simply crisscross your legs. If desired, take a few breaths to prepare.

2 Plant your palms on the floor beside your hips. Inhale and gaze forward.

3 As you exhale, brace your abdominal muscles and press into the floor with your hands as you begin to push upward. Think of pulling your lower and middle belly inward as you lift up.

4 Aim to hold for five full breaths, focusing on a gazing point, or *drishti*, in front of you. Imagine your stable core muscles keeping you lifted, balanced, and strong. Keep your palms anchored into the floor, pressing downward.

5 When you have held for as long as you can, release back down to the floor slowly and with control, keeping your gaze forward.

Take **1 minute** to explore the pose. Then, push up into Swing and hold for three full breaths, rest, and then repeat several more times for a total of **3 minutes**. If desired, try leaving the tips of your toes on the floor at first. Use your core strength, as well as your breath, to stay aloft in this gesture of both playfulness and strength.

In **12 minutes**, run through all of the poses in this lesson. Keeping your core engaged, notice how the poses challenge your core muscles in myriad ways. Tune into your areas of strength and weakness. As you hold your last Swing Pose, notice how your yogic core training is already impacting your energy levels, your powerhouse muscles, and your emotional state.

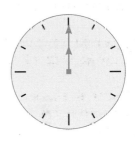

FIRE UP

Many yoga poses have the wonderful effect of imparting a potent burst of energy. In general, whenever a pose opens up the front of your body (think backbends, such as Camel Pose) or takes you into an inversion (like the pulse-quickening Shoulder Stand), you will feel energy enlivening your entire body from the inside out. Even if you are already feeling energetic, the poses in this section will help you to maintain these energy levels.

Complete this one-hour lesson, beginning with Breath of Fire and making your way through seven poses, and you will have a toolkit of invigorating yoga moves at your fingertips whenever you want a natural pick-me-up. Let your breath guide you through these poses. Keep breathing naturally as you become more and more energized.

Most of the poses in this section are part of the apex or height of a typical yoga class arc. But they can also be performed at intervals throughout the day, whenever you feel in need of natural invigoration.

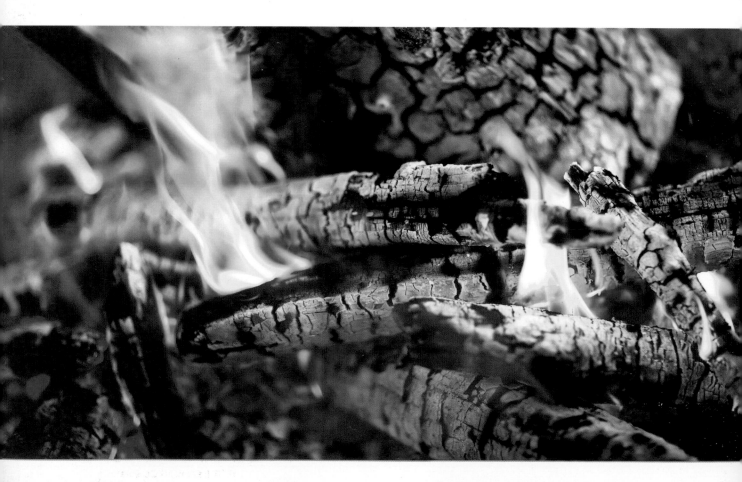

BREATH OF FIRE | BHASTRIKA PRANAYAMA

Breath of Fire is an energizing and cleansing breath that can literally fire you up from the inside out. Its Sanskrit name translates to "bellows breath"; practicing this breathing technique is akin to stoking a fire with bellows.

Benefits include waking up the body and mind by quickly oxygenating the blood, releasing toxins, easing anxiety, and lifting depression. This is a breathing exercise that demonstrates the sheer power and potency of your own breath. (Stop if you begin to feel dizzy or lightheaded at any point, and if you are menstruating or have high blood pressure it's best to skip this practice.)

1 Sit comfortably. Close your mouth gently, as you will be breathing through your nose. If you are just learning this breath, place one hand on your belly so that you can feel how it affects the core of your body.

2 Inhale and exhale once, naturally and fully.

3 Begin inhaling and exhaling more quickly, in short "sniffing" breaths. Typically your belly bulges outward as you exhale, but here, your belly should be moving inward on the exhalation instead. As you inhale and exhale rapidly, with equal duration, feel your belly moving.

4 Continue this pumping breath for several minutes. To finish, focus on the exhale, elongating it, for 3 deep breaths.

5 Sit for a few moments, breathing normally. Notice any changes in your mental and energetic state.

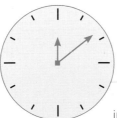

Run through this sequence, pumping your breath in step 4 for about **4 minutes**. Then complete step 4, lengthening your exhales for **1 minute**. Perform steps 4 and 5, and then resume normal breathing, noticing any changes in your energetic state, for **4 minutes**.

CHAIR POSE | UTKTASANA

Even if it initially seems a little awkward to sit in an imaginary seat, Chair Pose will impart a seriously energizing boost of power as it strengthens the powerhouse muscles of your core. Because this pose engages the large muscles of your legs, you'll most likely build heat quickly. Breathe through the heat as well as any shaking that may happen as your muscles get used to this position. As you lower into the imaginary chair, it is important to keep your alignment; your back should be neither arched nor rounded forward, and your shoulders should not be hunched but pressed down and away from your ears.

1 Stand upright, with your feet hip-width apart. Shift your weight slightly so that your weight rests on your heels.

2 Inhale, and raise your arms upward. Energize the arms all the way through your fingertips, which should be active and engaged. Allow your palms to face inward, and your fingers to spread wide.

3 Take a moment to engage your core. Think of pressing your navel toward your spine as you pull your abdominal muscles inward.

4 Tuck your tailbone. Bend your knees, and begin to slowly and smoothly lower yourself as if you were sitting down into an imaginary chair. At the same time, reach forward with your arms. Gaze in front of you.

5 Hold, taking full, deep breaths. Extend your fingers upward with each inhale.

EXTRA CREDIT Your thighs, buttocks, abdominals, and lower back muscles will benefit from this pose. Concentrate on keeping your core steady and stable to reap optimal strengthening benefits.

EXTRA CREDIT Focus on sitting back, not just down. To protect your knees, keep them aligned over your ankles. And to protect your lower back, focus on tucking your tailbone under rather than sticking your bottom outward.

Take **4 minutes** to explore Chair Pose, aiming to hold for about **30 seconds** each time, sitting deeper into the pose with every exhale. When releasing from the pose, inhale as you slowly straighten your legs. Then, gradually lower your arms to your sides.

Assume Chair Pose again—but this time, carry out Breath of Fire as you hold. Let the breath rev up your body and mind as you simultaneously feel grounded and solid in Chair. Allow **3 minutes**, releasing and repeating if necessary.

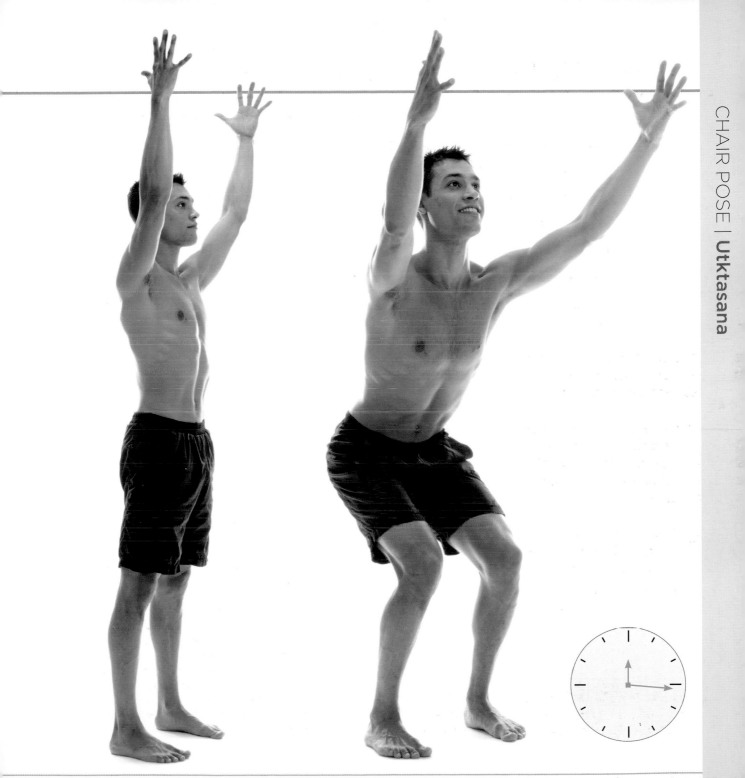

CAMEL POSE | USTRASANA

Camel Pose is an energizing, empowering heart opener. Sometimes this intense pose can make yogis a little dizzy; this is normal, so do your best to breathe through it. Of course, if the sensation feels intense, feel free to come back up and then sit on your heels in Hero's Pose (see page 123) for a few breaths. If you need extra padding under your knees you can to fold the mat once for support. For a deeper stretch, try resting the tops of your feet on the mat.

1 Kneel upright, with your knees hip-width apart. Bring your hands to your heart in a prayer position, and tuck your toes under.

2 Bring your hands to your lower back, fingers pointing down almost as if your fingers were resting in imaginary jeans pockets.

3 Inhale, lifting your chest up toward the ceiling. Exhale, tipping your head back. Bend through your upper, middle, and lower back. You can stop and hold here if desired.

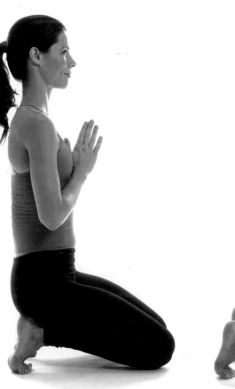

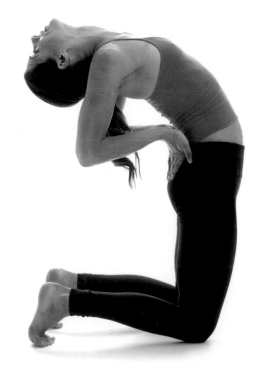

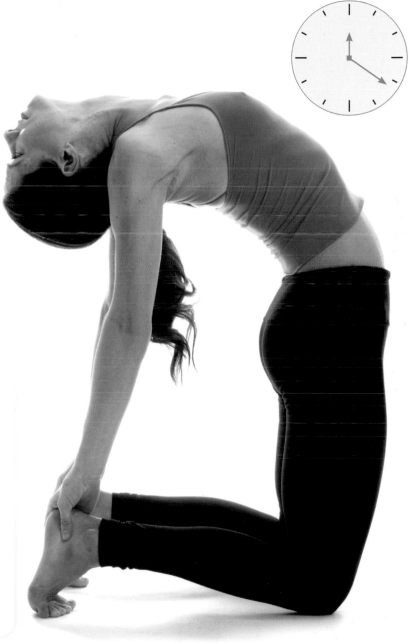

4 To deepen the pose, reach your hands to your heels. Imagine that there is an imaginary string on your heart pulling you upward as you push your hips forward. Hold for five breaths.

EXTRA CREDIT As you hold Camel Pose, press your hips forward and think about lifting up and out of the base of the spine rather than simply collapsing backward.

In **2 minutes**, complete steps 1 through 3, and then hold with your hands at your lower back. Notice the energizing feeling of opening at your heart and throat. Release, sitting straight up and forward.

Take about **30 seconds** to re-center yourself, bringing your hands to heart-center and noticing your heart beating against your thumbs—a bit more quickly than usual.

Take **3 minutes** to perform steps 1 through 4, and then hold. Release to sit upright, and again spend **30 seconds** re-centering yourself, bringing your hands to heart-center, and tuning in to your heartbeat against your thumbs.

BOW POSE | DHANURASANA

Bow Pose, sometimes called Floor Pose, stretches the entire front of your body, strengthens your back, and stimulates the organs of your abdomen. When you lift upward in step 3, your gaze is important; keep your eyes uplifted and your body will naturally follow. Feel your heart opening as you hold.

1 Lie facedown, resting your forehead on the mat.

2 Reach behind you with both hands, bend your knees, and reach around with your hands to grab your feet or ankles your feet from the outside.

3 Take a big breath in. Exhaling, kick your feet into your hands and lift your heels up and away. Gaze upward, toward the ceiling (taking care not to strain your neck).

4 Hold, breathing steadily. Even though you are on your stomach, pull your abdominal muscles inward as you feel your core growing stronger and tighter.

5 Exhale, releasing your feet from your hands and coming to rest on your stomach.

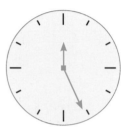

Spend **4 minutes** exploring the pose, holding in the full expression for a little longer each time. When you're done, exhale and release your feet from your hands, coming to rest on your stomach.

EXTRA CREDIT Bow Pose gives you a great opportunity to find your drishti, or gazing point. Keep your gaze uplifted and focus on an object in the room. Breathe in and out as you focus on this point and you will find this pose much easier hold. The uplifted feeling in your body will be easier to maintain, too.

SUPERHERO POSE

Superhero Pose is another energizing, invigorating pose that will engage your whole body, challenging your abs and your sense of balance. Its starting position, with both arms and legs extended, is a full pranam, or prostration, posture. Take a few breaths here to prepare if desired. Then, as you carry out the full pose, challenge yourself to lift higher and higher on each inhalation until you feel as powerful as a superhero soaring over a city.

1 Lie facedown. Your legs should be lengthened behind you, slightly pointed so that the tops of your feet face the floor. Your arms should be extended in front of you so that your whole body forms a straight line. Gaze forward.

2 Rest your forehead on the mat. Inhale to prepare. Take a big exhalation, breathing all of the air out of your body.

3 Inhale as you begin to lift your arms and legs upward. Raise them slowly and with control. The movement should be smooth, with no jerking motion.

4 Find your balance, keeping your gaze forward. Take three to five full breaths. On each inhalation, reach slightly higher. Go as high as you can without compromising your form or alignment.

5 On an exhalation, gradually lower your arms and legs. Lower them just as slowly as you lifted them, keeping your abs engaged throughout the movement.

EXTRA CREDIT As you begin to lift your arms and legs upward, try to use your abdominal muscles to drive the movement. Keep your core strong, active, and engaged.

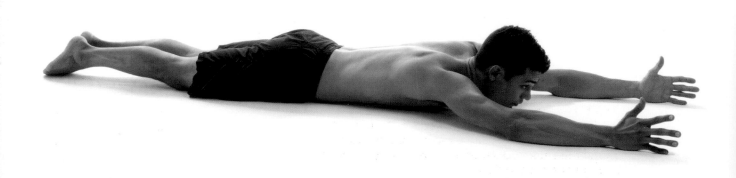

VARIATIONS

Harder
Bring your arms out to the side and back along your hips, with your palms facing downward. Keep your arms extended as you hold. This is called Full Locust.

EXTRA CREDIT
Do not allow your hips to tilt. Instead, keep them stable and square on your mat.

Carry out step 1, spending **30 seconds** anchoring your body into the floor in the full pranam.
Take **3 minutes** to explore the pose, including the harder variation. Finish by allowing one ear to rest on the mat. Take 30 seconds to listen to your heart beating against the floor.

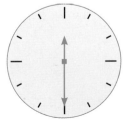

BRIDGE POSE | SETU BANDHASANA

Bridge Pose opens your chest and heart, tones your legs and glutes, and releases tension that you may be storing in your lower back. Just be sure to keep your head and neck straight to protect them from any stress of strain; looking to either side may tweak your neck. Your gaze should be upward as you assume the position and hold. You are always welcome to lift halfway rather than taking on the full expression of the pose right away. The beautiful thing about Bridge, also known as Half Wheel Pose, is that the extent to which you lift is up to you.

1 Lie on your back. Bend your knees to bring the soles of your feet onto the mat and plant them hip-width apart. Extend your arms along your sides. Allow your feet to stay planted on the mat, hip-width apart.

2 Empty all the breath out of the body. On an inhale, lift your hips high, keeping your shoulders on the floor. Press your hips toward the ceiling.

3 Interlace your fingers under your back—a hand position that allows you to push into the mat and lift your torso even higher. Walk your shoulders underneath your body and keep your arms straight, pressing into the mat as you lift your torso even higher.

4 Hold for three to five breaths. As you inhale and exhale, concentrate on keeping your torso completely steady, your abs pulled in, and your hips lifted. Your body from knees to shoulders should form a relatively straight line.

EXTRA CREDIT In starting position, reach down with your arms and see if you can brush the back of your ankles with your fingertips. If you can, then your alignment is correct.

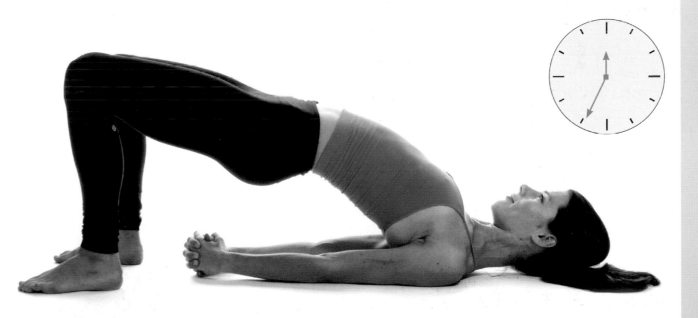

Allow yourself a full **4 minutes** to explore the pose step by step. Concentrate on the energizing sense of "opening up" the front of your body. (For a gentler version, try placing a yoga block beneath your lower back.) To release, remove your arms from under your torso and roll down, vertebra by vertebra.

FULL WHEEL POSE | URDHVA DHANURASANA

Full Wheel is a wonderful pose to take on after you've explored and feel comfortable in Bridge. Because it is so invigorating, some yogis avoid practicing it right before bed: it may give you too much energy and keep you up! It feels great in the morning or afternoon, however, when you need a pick-me-up. In fact, this pose opens up the entire front of the body, and is a wonderful expression of dropping the head below the heart and letting the heart lead. It is great for clearing the blues and lifting mild depression

1 Lie on your back with your knees bent and soles of the feet on the mat.

2 Reach down with your fingertips to check the alignment of the feet: they should be just far away from the bottom that your fingers can touch the heels.

3 Place your hands over your shoulders on the mat, next to your ears. Allow your fingertips to point toward your heels. Take a big breath in to prepare.

4 Exhale, pushing down into the floor with your feet and hands. Raise your entire torso toward the ceiling so that your body forms an upside-down U shape.

5 Hold for three to five breaths. With each breath, raise your torso higher.

For an extra-big boost of energy, take **7 minutes** to come into three consecutive Full Wheels. To release from each one, tuck your chin into your chest and slowly roll down. After finishing a three, counter the pose and release your lower back by squeezing your knees into your heart, again tuning into your heartbeat.

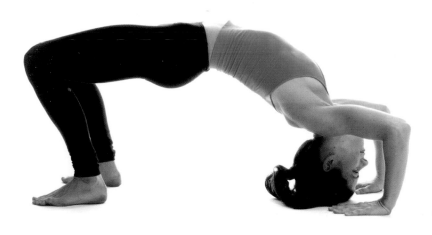

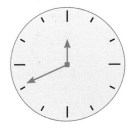

SHOULDER STAND | SALAMBA SARVANGASANA

Shoulder Stand is a safe and effective way to go upside down, giving you all the benefits that come with a yogic inversion. Beyond the fresh perspective this position will bring to your day, Shoulder stand stimulates the thyroid gland, calms the mind, and reduces fatigue. It is also an excellent toner for your legs and bottom.

1 Begin lying on your back. Rest your arms along your sides. Engage your core, activating your stomach muscles. Inhale to prepare.

2 Exhale as you begin to raise your legs toward the ceiling. Simultaneously, bend your elbows and "walk" your hands to your lower back. Your fingers should point toward your feet.

3 Hold for eight to ten breaths, sharpening your form with every breath. Your feet should be directly over your hips, your legs forming a straight line. Look up toward your feet.

Take **8 minutes** to explore Shoulder Stand, step by step. When holding, concentrate on the feeling of energy flowing through your entire body. Feel free to linger in Plow Pose as you come into or out of the inversion.

Release, and take **1 minute** to lie on your back, breathing naturally. Place your hands on your heart as you tune in to the energizing workout you've just performed.

Take **10 minutes** to run through the sequence of seven poses, from Chair Pose to Shoulder Stand. Hold Shoulder Stand for at least three full breaths before releasing.

VARIATIONS

Easier

Instead of extending your legs straight up toward the ceiling, try Plow instead. Often used as a preparatory pose for Shoulder Stand, Plow Pose is an inversion that is very effective for strengthening legs and back. Using your hands to support your lower back, bring your feet to the ground behind your head. Balance on your toes as you hold this pose. If you are having trouble with Shoulder Stand, or experience fear of falling over, begin with this pose. You can also come into Plow from Shoulder Stand to extend your energizing workout.

EXTRA CREDIT Make sure you are not holding tension in your neck and face as you hold Shoulder Stand. Soften your throat and relax your tongue.

TWIST YOURSELF FIT

When many people think of yoga, they envision stretching the body into pretzel-like shapes, like the arms and roots of an ancient tree. The following lesson will show you how to twist your body in myriad ways. Twists engage the right and left sides of the brain, invigorating both mind and body. Twists may also work to cleanse toxins from the organs as if you are wringing out your body as you would wring out a towel.

Some of the twists in this section include balance challenges. Other twists are more restorative and easy. There's a twisting pose for every body, every energy level, and every situation. Use your breath to guide you farther into the twisting shapes. Each exhale can release you deeper into your twist. Use your growing inner awareness to decide how far to twist today.

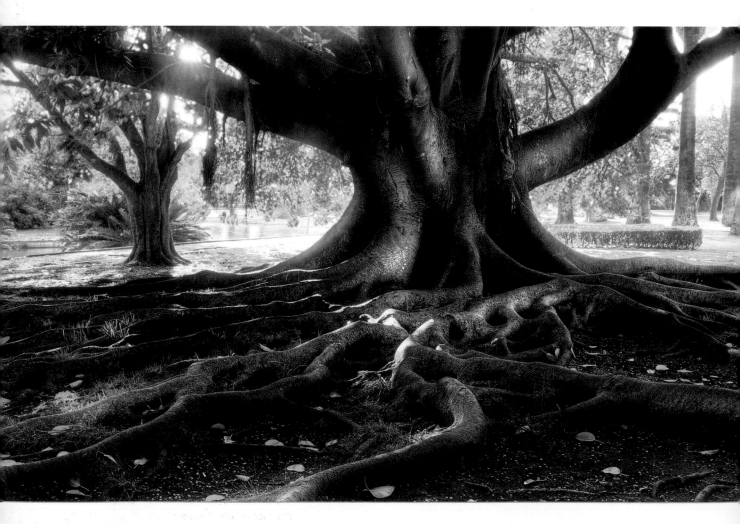

EAGLE POSE | GARUDASANA

Eagle Pose is probably the ultimate pose that combines balance with twisting. Here, you are squeezing toward the center of your body, engaging inward. Generally, the higher up you start the twist on the leg the better you will be able to twist. Don't worry if you can't achieve the double wrap, in either your arms or legs, right away. With practice, you will find yourself limbering up.

1 Stand in Mountain Pose (page 43). Inhale your arms high overhead.

2 Exhale, bending your elbows and twisting your right elbow under your left. See if you can achieve a double twist, at the elbows and wrists, bringing the hands to touch.

3 Press your legs together and sit down in an imaginary chair, making sure your knees are lined up over the ankles. Shift the weight into your left foot and raise your right leg, bringing your right knee over the left. You can try for the double wrap here, too, bringing the right foot behind the left ankle.

4 Stay in the shape for five breaths. While there, you can work to sit lower in your Eagle legs.

5 Release the shape on an exhale, extending all after such a big contraction. Repeat on the other side.

Spend **4 minutes** coming into this pose—on both sides. Experiment with your arm position: try raising your arm-shape so your upper arms are parallel to the floor before you begin to sit, and/or lower your elbows toward your knees as you hold.

REVOLVED HALF MOON | PARIVRTTA ARDHA CHANDRASANA

This is another pose that gives you a chance to balance—with a twist. As you take on the pose and then hold it, think of spiralling your torso upward from beneath your navel. Gaze is important; look downward and the pose feels easier, but look up toward your elevated hand and your sense of balance is challenged.

1 Begin in Standing Split (page 62) on your right leg, with the left leg extended. Position your fingertips on the floor, shoulder width apart.

Spend **4 minutes** exploring the pose. Move through all steps, on both sides. Keep breathing as you hold. With practice, you'll find your ability to hold this shape improving dramatically.

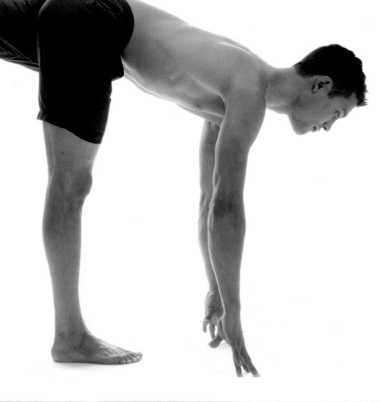

2 Bring your right hand to your right hip and begin to twist your chest open toward the right. Activate your left foot and reach your right hand upward toward the ceiling. Try to look at your right fingers. You are extended in a Half Moon shape while twisted.

3 Hold for five breaths before releasing. Repeat on the other side.

VARIATIONS

Easier
If you have trouble reaching the floor, place a block there and reach for it instead.

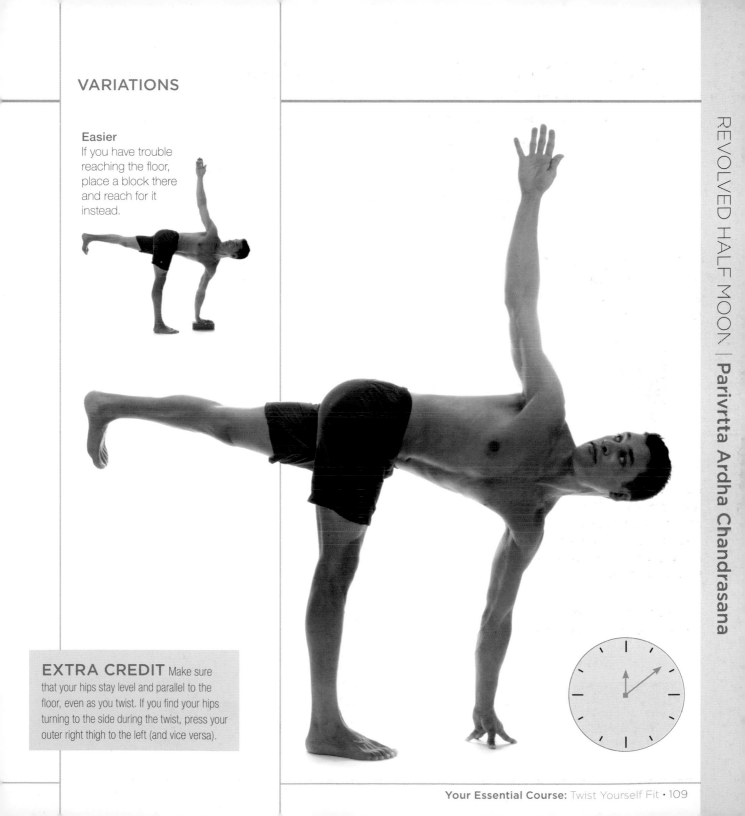

EXTRA CREDIT Make sure that your hips stay level and parallel to the floor, even as you twist. If you find your hips turning to the side during the twist, press your outer right thigh to the left (and vice versa).

THUNDERBOLT TWIST

Thunderbolt Twist feels restorative and energizing at the same time. As you hold, press your elbow into your knee to facilitate the turning upward of your heart-center upward. Think of spiraling your chest open, from below the belly button. Let your gaze find the ceiling.

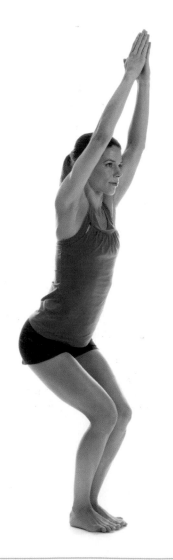

1 Stand in Mountain Pose (page 43). Bring your feet together so heels and toes touch.

2 Inhale your arms high overhead, looking at the thumbs, then exhale and sit back as if in a small chair, bringing the hands to heart-center.
This is Thunderbolt Pose.

3 Inhale, looking upward to create length. Exhale, twisting to the right. Hook your left elbow outside the right knee.

4 Hold for three to five breaths before releasing. Repeat on the other side.

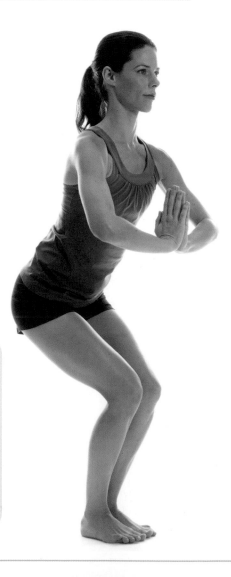

Take **2 minutes** to get to know this pose, step by step.
    Move on to a **3-minute** flow. Inhale in Thunderbolt Pose. Exhaling, twist to the left; inhaling, hold; exhaling, return to the center. Inhale. Exhaling, twist to the right; inhaling, hold; exhale, returning to the center again. Repeat, taking care not to rush the movement.

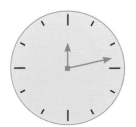

EXTRA CREDIT This pose targets those notoriously hard-to-reach oblique muscles. Concentrate on keeping your abdominal muscles stable, solid, and thoroughly pulled in. Do not allow them to bulge outward at any stage of the twist.

STANDING SPINAL TWIST | KATICHAKRASAN

Standing Spinal Twist is thought to help with detoxification of your abdominal organs. As you twist from the inside out, you will also stretch your back and release any tightness you may be holding in your chest area.

1 Assume a high lunge position. Tuck the toes of your back foot under, and bend your front knee so that your leg forms a 90-degree angle.

2 As you exhale, bring your arms downward in front of your body. Press your palms together in a prayer position. Position your hands at heart-center, in front of your upper chest.

3 Inhale and gaze upward, opening your chest. Exhale and twist so that your left elbow lands outside your right knee. Maintain your hand position as you twist. Gaze upward, over your right shoulder.

4 Challenge yourself to hold for eight to ten breaths. On each inhale, lengthen your spine; on each exhale, twist more deeply into the pose. Release, and then repeat on the other leg.

EXTRA CREDIT As you twist to the side and then hold the pose, be sure to keep your back leg activated and straight, from your hip to your toes. Imagine energy flowing all the way through to you back heel.

VARIATIONS

Harder

If you are breathing with ease in the twist, it is fine to move on. You can spread your arms wide apart like wings, coming into "fly away arms." Roll open your shoulders.

Easier

To make this pose slightly less strenuous, try performing it in a bound position. Bring your top arm behind your back and your bottom arm beneath the thigh of your front leg. Clasp your hands together and hold.

Take **6 minutes** to explore Standing Spinal Twist on both sides. Try both the harder and the easier variations, noticing which position feels most comfortable—and which challenges you in a satisfying way.

For **4 minutes**, carry out a twisting, balancing flow. Assume Thunderbolt Twist to the right side. Stay for a few breaths, and then step your left leg back into Standing Spinal Twist. Stay for a few breaths, and then step forward to Thunderbolt Twist. Repeat on the other side.

SEATED SPINAL TWIST | ARDHA MATSYENDRASANA

Seated Spinal Twist offers the opportunity to concentrate on the twisting position without having to focus on balance as well. Keep your abs engaged throughout the twist.

1 Sit upright with your legs crisscrossed. Pick up your right leg and bring it to the bring it to the outside of the left, using this moment to shift the left knee to a more central position. Allow the sole of the right foot to press into the mat.

2 Inhale your left arm up to the sky, then exhale, bringing the left elbow to the outside of the right knee. Let your right hand find the floor behind your back, tenting the fingertips.

3 Hold for three to five breaths. With each inhale raise the crown of your head higher, and with each exhale twist deeper, looking over the right shoulder.

4 Twist back to center. Repeat on the other side.

Take **4 minutes** to explore this pose on both sides. Free from the challenge of balance, focus on the twist in your abdomen and lower back.

VARIATIONS

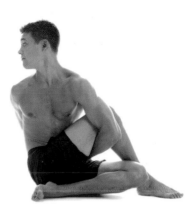

Easier

Try performing an easier version of the pose by taking on a bound position with your hands. Bring your left arm under your right thigh, and draw your right arm behind your back to meet your left. Grasp your hands and hold. Repeat on the other side.

EXTRA CREDIT This pose helps to strengthen and sculpt your abdomen. Like many other yoga twists, it offers great toning benefits for your oblique muscles. To reap these benefits, remember to keep your abdominal muscles active, engaged, and pulled inward.

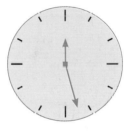

THREAD THE NEEDLE

Assuming twisting, winding shapes close to the floor are excellent, ironically, for *unwinding*. Thread the Needle is a calming cooling shape that is also a great shoulder opener. Keep your abs engaged and pulled in for an effective waist-whittling workout.

1 Begin on all fours. Inhale your left arm up toward the ceiling, then exhale, weaving the left hand under your right arm. Allow your left ear to rest on the mat. Your upper body is lowered in a twist with your hips remaining in the air as you stay on your knees.

2 Take three to five breaths in this shape, allowing your weight to sink into the mat.

3 Return to center and repeat on the other side.

EXTRA CREDIT
Thread the Needle helps to improve the range of motion and flexibility in your upper back and shoulders. In this way, it is a useful warmup exercise to perform before moving on to more challenging twists.

Spend **5 minutes** getting to know this pose. Imagine "melting" into the final shape, assuming a position of both strength and passivity as your upper body twists.

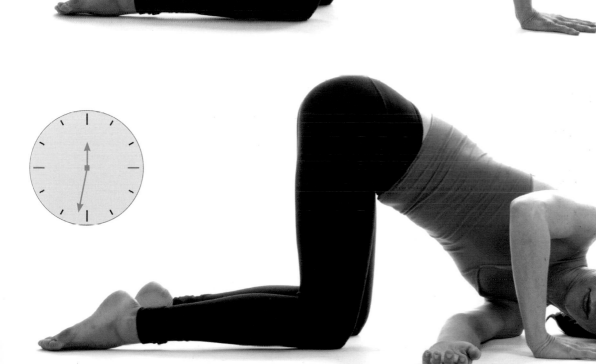

COMPASS POSE | PARIVRTTA SURYA YANTRASANA

Compass Pose combines many different stretches into one beautiful shape. As you hold the pose, you are stretching the entire side of your body, especially your hip and shoulder. Over time, you will be able to stretch farther and farther into this advanced shape. With time your leg and hip will be able to open up more fully.

1 Sit upright, with your legs crisscrossed and your back tall. Bring your left foot to the floor so that your knee points upward.

2 Lift your left leg with your right hand, grasping the outside edge of the foot for a sturdy grip. Plant your left palm into the floor. Position your upper arm beneath the crook of your knee or hamstring. Your elbow will be bent, making a "shelf" of your upper arm.

3 Exhale and begin extending your left leg by kicking your left foot into your right hand. At the same time, spiral your chest upward and to the side, raising your arm and looking under your right shoulder toward the ceiling. Hold for five to eight breaths. Then, release and repeat on the other side.

EXTRA CREDIT
As you learn the pose, feel free to pause along the way. Any step of Compass is a great place to be.

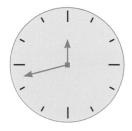

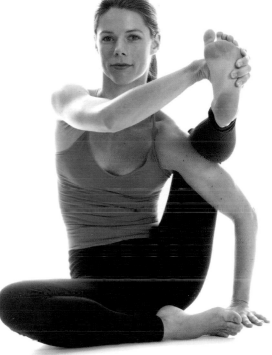

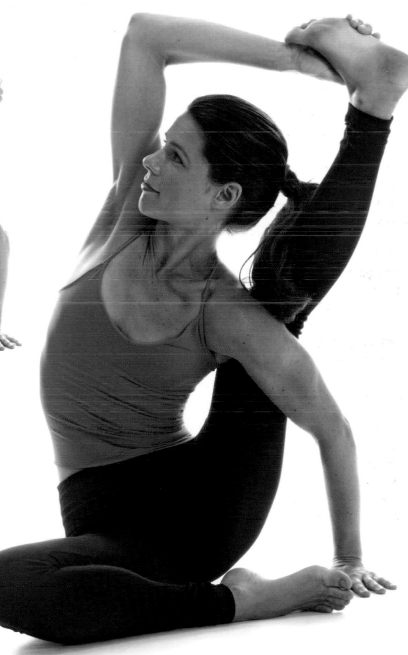

Allow **6 minutes** to explore this stretching twist on both sides. Notice how your stretching ability changes, even during this short period.

Perform Seated Spinal Twist, Thread the Needle, and then Compass Pose to the right side, and then run through all three on the left side, taking a total of **5 minutes** to thoroughly stretch your lower abdomen, your upper abdomen, and both sides of your body respectively.

FULL LOTUS POSE | PADMASANA

Full Lotus Pose is a classic yoga position many are familiar with. There are many steps and variations of this pose. Remember that no two bodies are alike and due not just to body type but bone structure, some parts of Lotus pose may be easier for some yogis than for others. Full Lotus pose naturally positions the body so the hips are above the knees. You can also find this base position by sitting cross-legged with a folded blanket or pillow under your sit bones. With the hips elevated above the knees, the spine stays more naturally straight for seated meditation.

1 Sit upright, with your arms down by your sides, palms on the floor. Your legs should be extended in front of you.

2 Bend your right knee and open it up to the side. Lower your right thigh to the floor as your right hip begins to open.

3 Bend your left knee and bring it toward your body. Crisscross your legs so you are now sitting upright with legs crossed. Bring your hands to rest on your knees, palms facing up. Your hips should now be open. Gaze forward.

4 Using your hands if desired, bring your right foot on top of your left thigh, positioning it so that the top of the foot rest on the thigh and the sole of the foot faces the ceiling. This is Half Lotus.

5 Bring your left foot to rest on top of the right thigh. Hold for five to eight breaths, or longer if you are meditating. Release, and then repeat on the other leg if desired.

EXTRA CREDIT Yogis believe that the ability to sit and meditate is a reward to be gleaned from yoga practice. Whether you sit with your breath and your thoughts for three breaths, allow your time in this Full Lotus Pose to serve as your reward.

Give yourself **2 minutes** to explore the steps to Full Lotus Pose—on both sides.

Take **15 minutes** to move through all of the twists in this lesson, performing them on both sides where appropriate. At the end, linger in Full Lotus, breathing meditatively as you let the twisting you have just performed resonate throughout your body and mind.

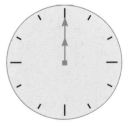

MOONLIGHT WIND-DOWN

Yoga is the perfect nightcap. At the end of a long day, many yoga practices and poses are at our disposal to help us wind down. The poses in this lesson calm the mind and the nervous system, allowing you to breathe deeply, let go of tension, and and prepare for restful sleep.

As you practice the following poses, take long, full breaths and allow your body to release. Let yourself linger. As you wind down, the goal is to let the yoga work on you rather than the other way around. As you inhale and exhale, focus on receive the benefits that each pose has to offer.

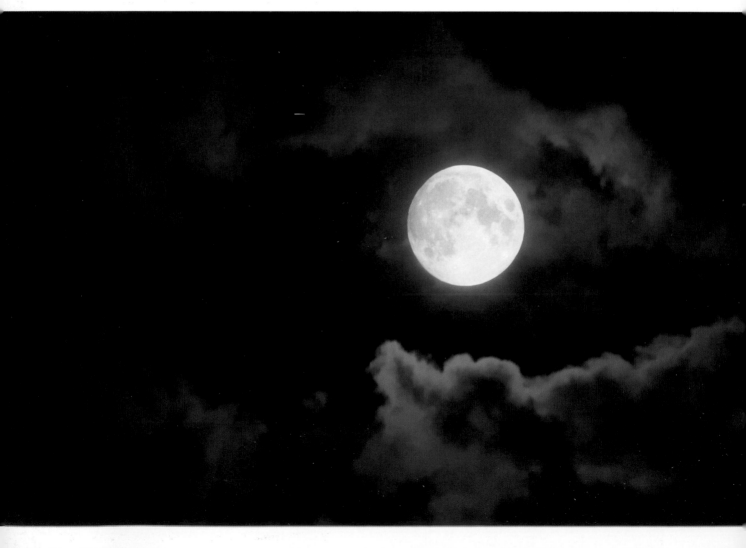

HERO POSE | VIRASANA

Hero Pose will give you a feeling of stability. While holding this pose, tune into your breath as you notice a sense of openness and steadiness pervading your body and mind. If the pose feels too intense on your knees, try sliding a folded blanket beneath them. Hero Pose is a valuable counter to hip-opening poses such as Full Lotus.

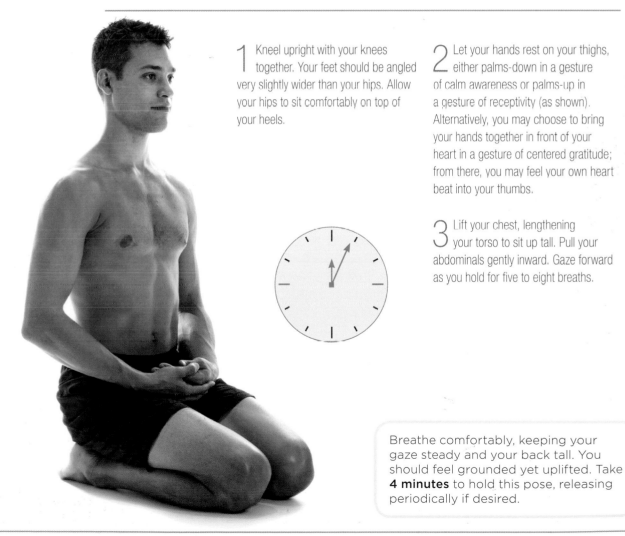

1 Kneel upright with your knees together. Your feet should be angled very slightly wider than your hips. Allow your hips to sit comfortably on top of your heels.

2 Let your hands rest on your thighs, either palms-down in a gesture of calm awareness or palms-up in a gesture of receptivity (as shown). Alternatively, you may choose to bring your hands together in front of your heart in a gesture of centered gratitude; from there, you may feel your own heart beat into your thumbs.

3 Lift your chest, lengthening your torso to sit up tall. Pull your abdominals gently inward. Gaze forward as you hold for five to eight breaths.

> Breathe comfortably, keeping your gaze steady and your back tall. You should feel grounded yet uplifted. Take **4 minutes** to hold this pose, releasing periodically if desired.

SEATED FORWARD FOLD | PASCHIMOTTANASANA

As you hold Seated Forward Fold, the magic comes from releasing. This pose will strengthen your hamstrings, back, and shoulders. Beyond these physical benefits, it provides an excellent way to unwind, calming the mind and reducing stress.

1 Sit upright, with your legs extended long in front of you. Bring your legs together as if they were a single leg. Flex your feet so that your toes point back toward your body.

2 Take a moment to rock from side to side to sit more directly on your sit bones, noticing your alignment.

3 Inhale, sitting up tall and raising your arms overhead. Extend your arms so that they stretch as far overhead as possible.

4 Exhale, feeling a sense of release as you bend from your hips and fold your upper body forward and then down over your legs. At the same time, bring your extended arms down over the front of your body and reach for your toes, grasping them your hands if possible. Inhale, lengthening your spine.

Explore this pose for **4 minutes** as you hold, releasing if necessary before adopting the pose instead. Enjoy the sensation of release, coupled with intense stretch.

5 Exhale and fold deeper into the pose, gradually lowering your upper body. Aim to rest your upper torso on top of your thighs while resting your elbows on the floor.

6 Gaze downward, relaxing your head and neck. Release your shoulders. Imagine drawing your heart forward as you hold for eight to ten full breaths before releasing.

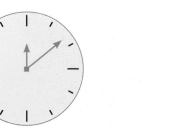

EXTRA CREDIT Before bringing your arms upward, try rocking from side to side on your sit bones. This will help you to rest on top of them more directly, augmenting the stability of Seated Forward Fold.

BUTTERFLY POSE | BADDHA KONASANA

The meditative Butterfly Pose will help you to relax and tune into how your body and mind are feeling at the end of your yoga practice. Let your knees flop open toward the floor as you breathe further and further into the stretch. Beyond its relaxation benefits, Butterfly Pose provides an excellent stretch for your inner thighs.

1 Sit upright. Bring the soles of your feet together so that they are touching, and draw the heels toward your groin.

2 Gently open up the soles of your feet as if you were opening the pages of a book. Rock back and forth on the sit bones to find your most stable seat and tallest extension. Let your knees "butterfly" open. Remain in this position if desired.

3 Hinging at the hips, fold gradually forward. Leading with the heart, fold the upper body first forward and then down in a release.

4 Continue to lower your upper body, bending your arms until your elbows rest on your legs. Hold for five to eight breaths, and then release.

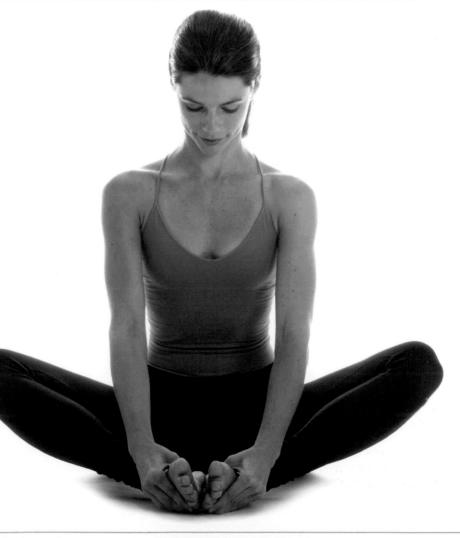

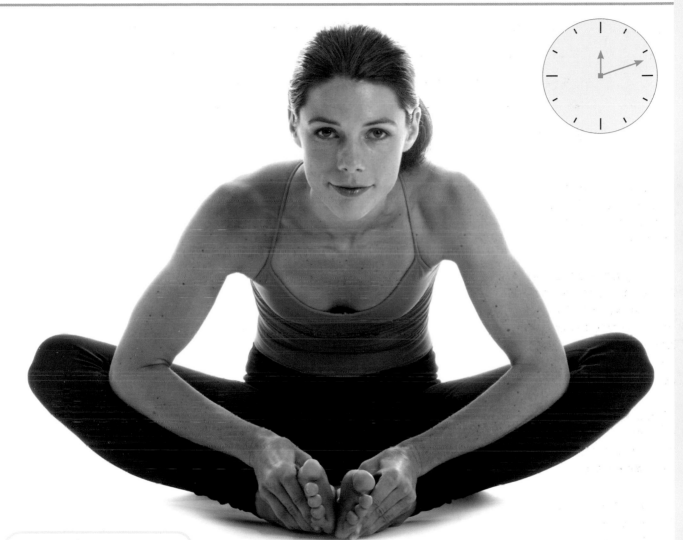

As with Seated Forward Bend, relax into Butterfly Pose while undertaking a powerful stretch at the same time. For **4 minutes**, hold the pose, resting periodically if desired.

HAPPY BABY POSE | ANANDA BALASANA

Happy Baby is a highly effective hip stretch. Babies really do take on this pose, and look very happy doing it! See if you can come into this naturally joyful pose with a sense of letting go. As you breathe through the pose, try rocking from side to side. Flutter through the lips to release the muscles of your face. Feel free to rock from side to side, enjoying the openness of the shape and massaging your back against your mat.

1 Lie face-up on the floor. Inhale to prepare. On an exhalation, bend your knees and draw your legs toward your chest. Grasp your knees with your arms.

2 Grasp your ankles with both hands. Position your feet so that the soles face the ceiling. Take another inhalation to prepare.

3 Exhaling, begin to straighten your legs, extending them upward. Continue to hold your ankles in your hands. Using your hands, draw your feet apart to open your legs.

4 Hold for eight to ten breaths, continuing to gently pull your feet wider apart and down toward the floor with every breath. Feel free to rock from side to side if desired; after all, this pose is meant to be fun! The rocking motion will help to release any tension you may be storing in your hips.

5 On an exhalation, release your grip on your ankles and slowly bring your feet back to the floor.

Here's your chance to really let go. Allow yourself **3 minutes** to explore this pose, rocking on the floor as you say goodbye to the day's stress— and the tension it may be causing in your body and mind.

Take **3 minutes** to go through Hero, Butterfly, Seated Forward Fold, and then Happy Baby, holding each for as long as you feel is necessary. Devote this sequence to focusing inward, noticing any tension you may be harbouring in the form of hunched shoulders, stifled breathing, et cetera. As much as possible, let go of that tension.

CAT TO COW | MARJARYASANA TO BITILASANA

Both Cat Pose and Cow Pose are highly effective for warming up your spine and stretching your back. But beyond benefiting your back, moving back and forth between these poses with conscientious breathing invigorates your whole body and your mind as well. Try this whenever you have a few minutes to spare.

1 Kneel on all fours, with your shoulders aligned over your wrists and your knees and hips stacked. Pull your abdominal muscles inward towards your spine and assume a flat back. Look downward so that your neck is neutral. Inhale to prepare.

2 Exhale, arching your back like a Halloween cat. Pull your navel inward, imagining pressing it toward your spine and let your head and hips drop.

3 Inhale directly into Cow, leting your belly drop and your chest expand. Shift your gaze upward. Both your tailbone and your head will be arching upward while your midsection sways and releases.

4 Exhale, coming back into Cat. Move back into step 3 if desired.

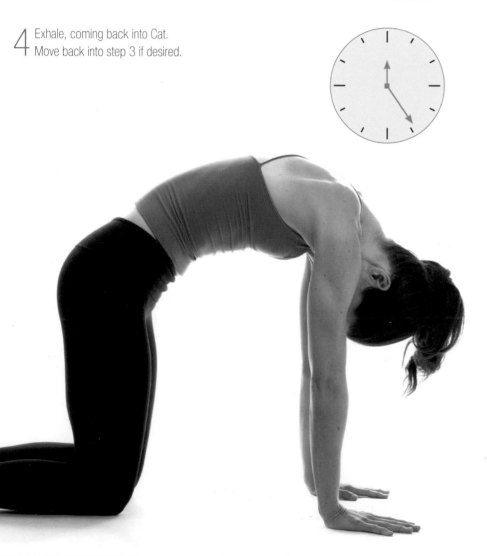

EXTRA CREDIT Keep your movement smooth and controlled as you transition between the two poses. Avoid any sort of jerking motion.

Spend **2 minutes** learning Cat to Cow, step by step. Then, spend **2 minutes** moving from Cat to Cow and back again, with no pauses in between. Keep your motion smooth, guided by your breath. Allow a further **2 minutes** to improvise in both the Cat and the Cow positions; try circling your hips and/or shoulders, releasing any tension that you feel in your upper body, back, or neck.

CHILD'S POSE | BALASANA

Child's Pose is a gesture of rest and recovery. In a typical yoga class, students are invited to assume the pose whenever they need a moment to reconnect to their breath. This pose slows the heart rate and rests the whole body and the mind. Feel the connection between your forehead and the mat. It's nice to close your eyes in this pose and relax the muscles of your face. There is no one "correct" way to carry out Child's Pose; choose the variation that feels right for you on any given day. This choosing is a practice of intuition. Listen to your body and do what feels right in the moment.

1 Kneel upright, with your hips on top of your heels.

2 Fold your upper body forward until your forehead is resting on your mat.

3 Extend your arms behind your body, palms up so that the tops of your hands face the floor.

4 Take three to five breaths here, staying longer if desired.

EXTRA CREDIT Try to tune in to any stress that you may be carrying in your shoulders. Take a moment to hunch your shoulders, and then release them. Picture them relaxing into the floor, widening all the way across your upper back and pulling away from your ears. Let your neck relax, too; it should be neither arched nor curved forward as your forehead releases downward. Feel free to close your eyes to enhance the sensation of letting go.

VARIATIONS

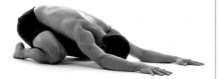

Same Level of Difficulty
Separate your upper legs, allowing your torso to spill into the space between them to rest on the floor. Extend your arms in front of you and rest them on the floor, palms down.

Here's your chance to rest and look inward. Remain in Child's Pose for about **5 minutes**, breathing deeply and heavily. Look for a feeling of restoration. Try the variation and notice which feels best to you.

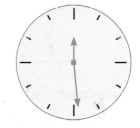

PIGEON POSE | EKA PADA KAPOTASANA

Pigeon Pose opens up your hips in a big way. After a day spent sitting at a desk or in the car—or walking around the city in high heels!—taking a few minutes for Pigeon will feel incredible. It is best to stay in this shape for as many breaths as possible to reap as much benefit as possible. It is important to let go: the more you release the more you will feel the benefits of Pigeon. Be gentle with your joints. Fold forward as deeply as is comfortable, but back out of the stretch if you feel any pain.

1 Assume Downward-Facing Dog (page 52). Inhale and raise your right leg behind you, keeping it energized and extended.

2 Exhale and bring the leg forward, in between your hands. Rest the foot on the floor, bent so that your knee is positioned outside of your right elbow. Position your right shin as parallel to the front of the mat as possible. Keep your left leg straight, extended behind you with the foot resting on the mat.

3 Inhale, raising your upper chest and gazing toward the ceiling. Take a moment to acknowledge a sense of openheartedness. Come up onto your fingertips in preparation for folding forward.

4 Exhale, folding forward and then down to rest your torso over your front leg. Keep your forehead down so the back of your neck stays straight. Hold for eight to ten breaths. Then, release and repeat on the other side.

EXTRA CREDIT Yogis sometimes report that unexpected feelings arise while performing Pigeon, as the hips are thought to hold memories and emotions. Breathe through any sensations that you may feel.

More than any other pose in this lesson, Pigeon is challenging. In fact, it can be very intense. Give yourself **3 minutes** to explore the pose, step by step, on both sides. Challenge yourself to hold for a long period: **4 minutes** on one side, and then **4 minutes** on the other. Keep your hips square. Attempt the harder variation if you feel comfortable doing so.

Then, go through all of the poses in this lesson, from Hero onward, remaining in each as long as you feel comfortable. Allow a full **12 minutes**.

VARIATIONS

Harder

Stay upright in the Pigeon shape, bend the back knee and hook your back foot with your elbow or grab it with the hand (on the same side as the foot). This will bring a quadriceps stretch into Pigeon. Think of opening the chest and gazing upward.

CORPSE POSE | SAVASANA

Corpse pose is often said to be one of the most important poses of yoga. We practice this pose at the end of a yoga session to allow the body, mind, and spirit to integrate all the poses that came before in practice. Though it may look like simply lying on the floor and resting, it is a pose just like any other.

1 Lie down on your mat, allowing your feet to flop open and your arms to separate, palms up. You can think of your body flopping open symmetrically from its center line. Close your eyes and allow your breath to be soft. Feel your body to be heavy and your mind light.

2 If there is still some tension in the body you may way to do a quick body scan, encouraging any tense places to relax and release. You can even move through the body part by part, beginning at the toes and working your way up to the head, encouraging each part to tense on the inhale then release on the exhale.

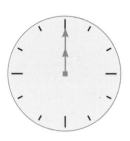

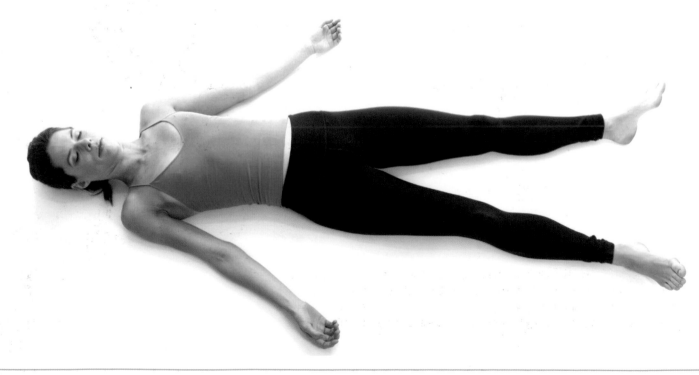

3 Hold Corpse Pose. Breathe normally, and imagine your mind becoming light and your body heavy. When it's time to come out of it, roll onto your right side for a breath or two, resting in a fetal position shape. At this moment, you are moving from the corpse pose to the fetal position in a physical reminder of rebirth, of a new moment.

4 When you are ready to sit up, press the left hand into the ground and push up to sit in a comfortable, cross-legged position. Take a few more breaths.

Breathe deeply and meditatively as you hold pose for **7 minutes**. Allow **1 minute** to gradually emerge from Corpse Pose.

EXTRA CREDIT Close your eyes. This pose is all about release. Try to relax any remaining tension in the body and the mind. Let your body melt into the floor; the more you let go, the more the floor can support you here. Let your mind float and let your breath be soft. Let your body, mind, and spirit absorb all of the benefits of your yoga practice.

CORPSE POSE | **Savasana**

HOW TO ACE A STUDIO CLASS

Now that you're learning all about yoga and trying it at home, you may want to consider taking a class! Studio yoga classes offer a great opportunity to practice with others; often, simply being in a room with fellow yogis who are focusing, breathing, and stretching can give your own yoga practice a supportive boost.

If you are new to yoga class, consider arriving a little early and introducing yourself to the teacher. You may want to mention that you are new to the studio yoga experience, and if you are working with any injuries or special situations (whether physical, mental, or emotional), you are welcome to let the teacher know. Teachers are there to guide and support.

Remember: Your yoga practice is your own. During class, all instructions in yoga are actually more like invitations. If something hurts or doesn't feel right in your body, it is all right to carry out a variation on your own, or even to rest in Child's Pose. In fact, when your body is telling you to do so, assuming Child's Pose—rather than pushing through something that isn't right for you—can be very empowering. Remaining tuned in to your own body's signals in the face of pressure is, after all, an advanced practice.

During the session, your teacher may give you physical adjustments which are usually meant to guide you deeper into the poses. For example, he or she may gently press on your lower back during Child's Pose to help you take on a deeper stretch than you may otherwise achieve. Adjustments may also be suggested if you are out of alignment in a way that carries a risk of injury. If you would rather not be adjusted physically during your class, simply let the teacher know before the session begins.

Most studios have their own mats, blocks, straps, and supplies, but you are welcome to bring your own if desired. And if you are more comfortable being in the back of the class at first, that is fine. Often it's nice to be in the back when you are new to the studio experience, so that you can peek at more experienced practitioners in the front if you get confused.

However, try to resist constant comparisons with others. While it is fine to peek at someone's else's form when you're just learning where a knee or foot should go, remind yourself that yoga is not a competitive sport. Everyone in the room is doing their best as they discover what suits their individual needs; yoga students tend to be tuned in to their own practice, rather than (for instance) measuring the extent of your stretches.

Every yoga teacher is different, and so many different studios and styles are available. As you venture out to explore yoga classes, keep in mind that if you don't love one you are free to try another. Not every instructor is right for everyone, and certain styles resonate better with certain people than with others. You may even notice that different yoga practices appeal to you during different periods of your life; even if you desire a vigorous practice now, next year you might crave something more restorative. This is part of yoga practice, too: everything changes. Try to go with the flow. As long as you stay curious, receptive, and non-judgmental (of yourself, above all) you will ace your yoga experience—in the living room, the studio, or wherever your practice takes you.

III. WORK IT OUT

Now that you have learned how to perform some essential yoga poses, you are ready to put them together in a variety of flows. No matter how pressed for time you may be, you can still reap the benefits of yoga practice—and these workouts prove it. Whether you are looking to target a particular body part, cultivate a certain mental or emotional state, or address something that ails you, there is likely to be a combination of yoga poses to take you there. Each workout lasts roughly 15 to 20 minutes, except for Yoga Fixes for Busy People (see page 152) which each take between 2 and 8 minutes to complete. Of course, you can modify these workouts by holding the poses for longer or shorter durations, building in repetitions of certain sequences or skipping any parts that do not feel especially beneficial. And feel free to create your own yoga flows using what you've learned throughout your Essential Course. Just one rule applies to all of these quick workouts: stay connected to your breath at all times. And be sure to give yourself some time for Corpse Pose. Relaxing at the end of a yoga workout allows all of the benefits to sink into your body, mind, and spirit.

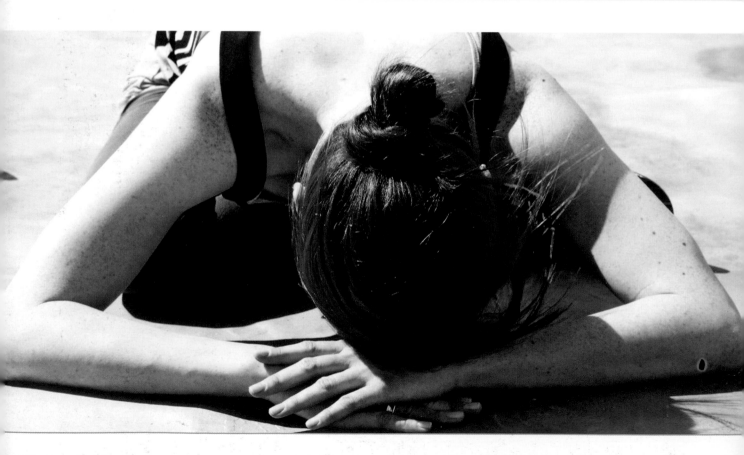

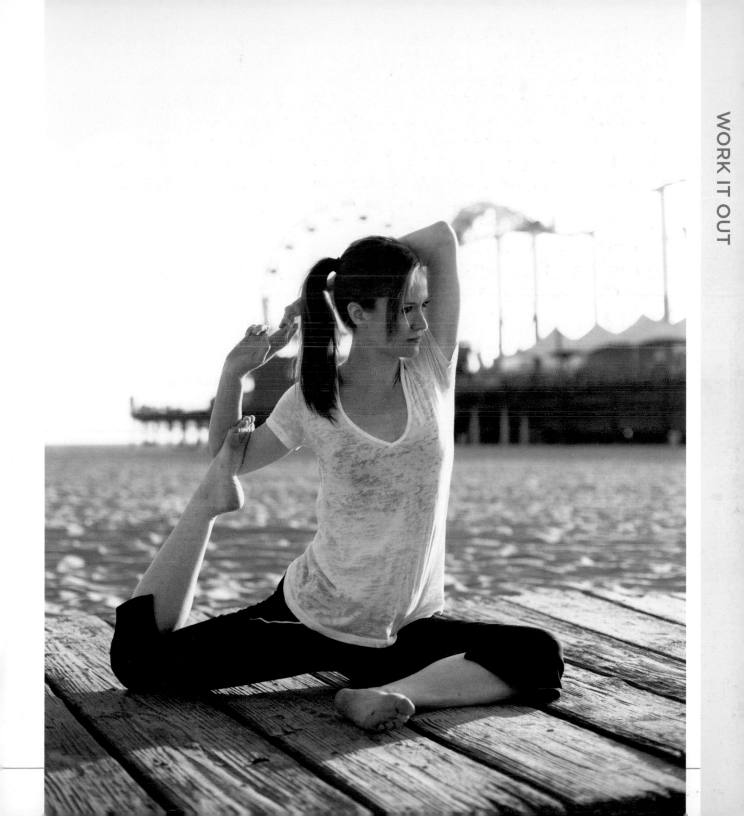

SUN SALUTATIONS

Sun Salutations A and B are classic flows and great additions to your yoga repertoire. Make sure to alternate the sides on which you perform certain poses, such as Warrior I. Move with the breath, allowing each movement to correspond with an inhale or exhale. Sun Salutations warm up all of the body, making them good low-impact cardiovascular workouts. Use your breath to reinforce your sense of connectedness between your body and mind.

SUN SALUTATION A

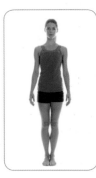

1. Mountain Pose

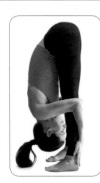

2. Forward Fold

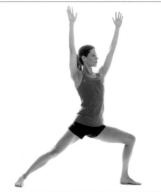

3. Warrior I

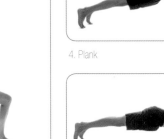

4. Plank

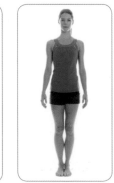

5. Chaturanga

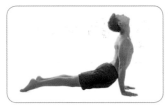

6. Upward-Facing Dog

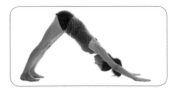

7. Downward-Facing Dog (hold for 5 breaths)

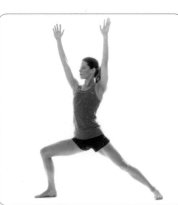

8. Warrior I (left leg back)

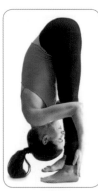

9. Forward Fold

10. Mountain Pose

SUN SALUTATION B

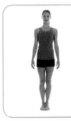

1. Mountain Pose

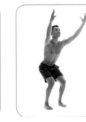

2. Chair Pose

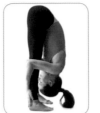

3. Forward Fold

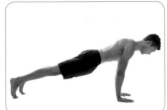

4. Plank

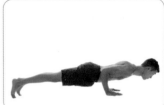

5. Chaturanga

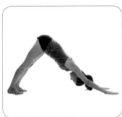

6. Downward-Facing Dog

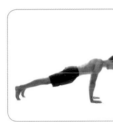

7. Warrior I

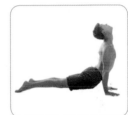

8. Plank

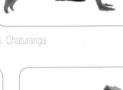

9. Chaturanga

10. Upward-Facing Dog

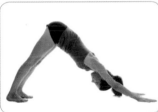

11. Downward-Facing Dog

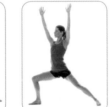

12. Warrior I

13. Plank

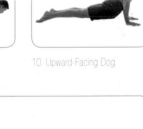

14. Chaturanga

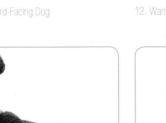

15. Upward-Facing Dog

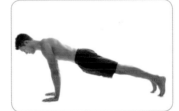
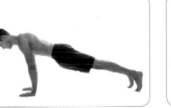

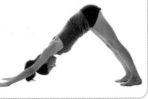

16. Downward-Facing Dog (hold for 3–5 breaths, then bend knees, look forward, and step between hands)

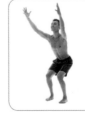

17. Forward Fold

18. Chair Pose

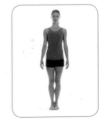

19. Mountain Pose

YOGA 24/7

While it is great to have a spare hour or two to dedicate to a full yoga practice, the great thing about yoga is that's it is flexible. Even 15 minutes on the yoga mat can drastically change how you feel. Squeezing in a quick workout in the morning, again at noon, and then in the evening is a wonderful way to stay connected to body and breath throughout the day. Honor the differences in how you feel throughout the course of a day by exploring these routines.

MORNING PUMP-UP

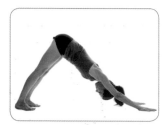

1. Child's Pose (hold for 5 deep breaths)

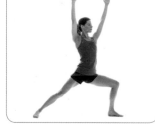

2. Cat to Cow (perform 5 repetitions)

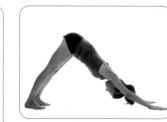

3. Thread the Needle (hold for 5 breaths, and then repeat on the other side)

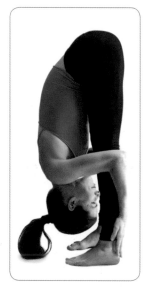

7. Forward Fold (hold for 3–5 breaths)

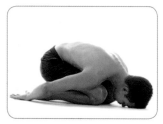

4. Downward-Facing Dog (hold for 5 breaths)

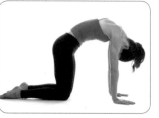

5. Warrior I (hold for 3 breaths, and then repeat on the other side)

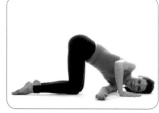

6. Downward-Facing Dog (hold for another 5 breaths)

AFTERNOON BREAK

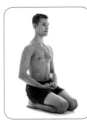

1. Hero's Pose (hold for 5 deep breaths)

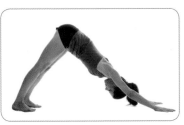

2. Downward-Facing Dog (hold for 5 deep breaths)

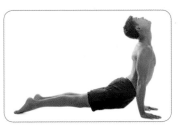

3. Sun Salutation A (perform twice, at a relaxed pace)

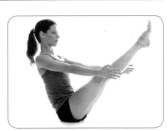

4. Boat Pose (hold for 5 breaths; try variations if desired)

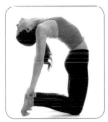

5. Camel (hold for 5 breaths)

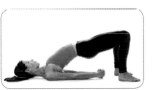

5. Bridge Pose (hold for 5 breaths)

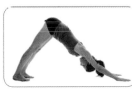

6. Knees to Chest (hold for 5 breaths)

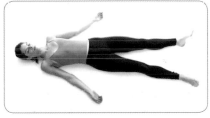

7. Corpse Pose (hold for 10 deep breaths)

EVENING ZEN

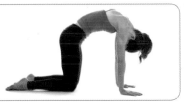

1. Cat to Cow (hold for 2 breaths each, and then repeat)

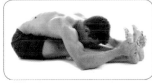

2. Seated Forward Fold (hold for 5 breaths)

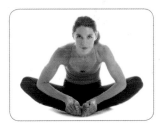

3. Butterfly (hold for 5 breaths)

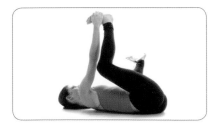

4. Happy Baby (hold for 5 breaths)

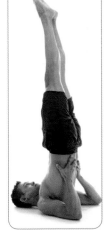

5. Shoulder Stand (hold as long as possible, breathing comfortably)

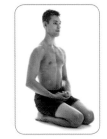

6. Hero's Pose (hold for 2 minutes, trying Alternate-Nostril breathing)

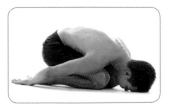

7. Child's Pose (hold for at least 10 deep breaths)

THE YOGI'S CHALLENGE

The following sequences will challenge you take on shapes that may look daunting at first. With practice, you will prove to yourself that you can do far more than you thought you could! Follow these sequences when you are feeling especially daring in order to push your limits and transcend your comfort zone, both physically and mentally.

ADVANCED SEQUENCE 1

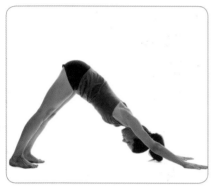

1. Downward-Facing Dog (hold for 3–5 breaths)

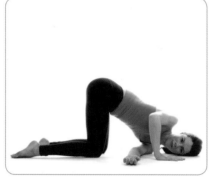

2. Thread the Needle (hold for 5–8 breaths, and then repeat on the other side)

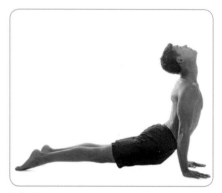

3. Sun Salutation A (perform twice, with 1 breath per movement)

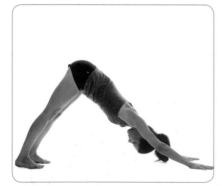

4. Downward-Facing Dog (hold for 5 breaths)

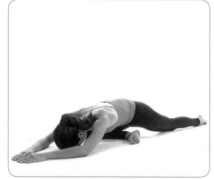

5. Pigeon (hold for 5–8 breaths, and then repeat on the other side)

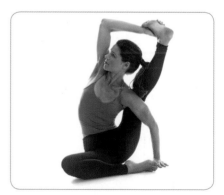

6. Compass Pose (both sides)

ADVANCED SEQUENCE 2

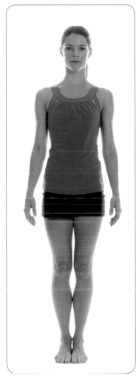

1. Mountain Pose (while holding, roll shoulders a few times)

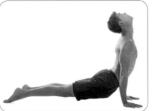

2. Sun Salutation A (perform twice, with 1 breath per movement)

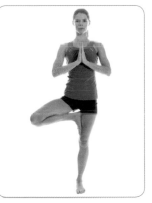

3. Tree Pose (hold for 5 breaths, and then repeat on the other side)

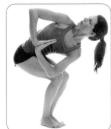

4. Thunderbolt and Thunderbolt Twist (both sides)

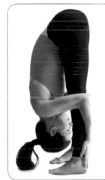

5. Forward Fold

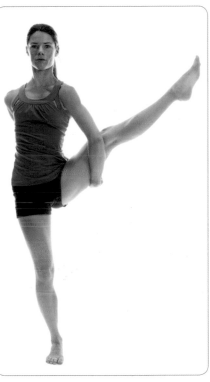

6. Bird of Paradise

ADVANCED SEQUENCE 3

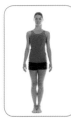

1. Mountain Pose

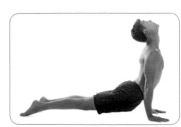

2. Sun Salutation A (perform 3 times, with 1 breath per movement)

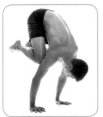

3. Chair Pose

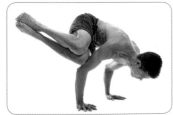

4. Crow Pose

5. Side Crow Pose

FIRING UP

Who needs coffee? Fire up your body the natural way by incorporating the following sequences into your day. These sequences strengthen major muscle groups, including the core muscles, and invigorate your body. What's more, you will come away from these flows with a greatly improved ability to focus.

These routines create heat within the body and encourage you to lighten up; after all, there's no need to carry around anything you don't need. Let your tension—and calories—burn away as you grow stronger and leaner with regular practice. For extra energy, you may wish to preface these sequences with three rounds of Breath of Fire (page 91).

FIRE UP SEQUENCE 1

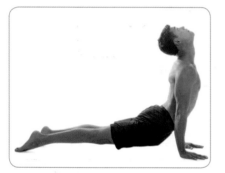

1. Sun Salutation A (perform 3 times, with 1 breath per movement)

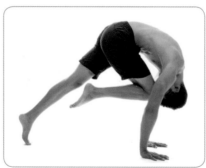

2. Knee to Nose (perform 3 repetitions)

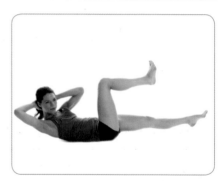

3. Yoga Bicycles (1 breath per movement, working up to 20 breaths)

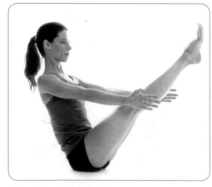

4. Boat Pose (perform 3–5 repetitions)

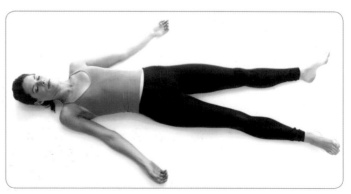

5. Corpse Pose (hold for 1 minute or longer)

FIRE UP SEQUENCE 2

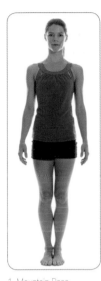

1. Mountain Pose

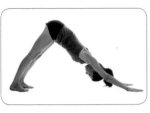

2. Sun Salutation B (perform 3 times, with 1 breath per movement)

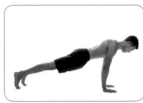

3. Plank (hold for 8–10 breaths)

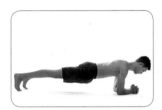

4. Forearm Plank (hold for 5–8 breaths)

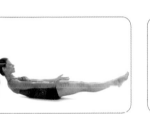

5. Boat to Half Boat (1 breath per movement; perform 10 repetitions)

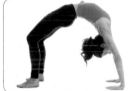

6. Full Wheel Pose (hold for 5–8 breaths; perform 1 repetition, working up to 3)

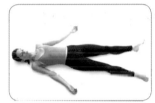

7. Corpse Pose (hold for 1 minute or longer)

FIRE UP SEQUENCE 3

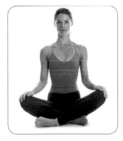

1. Sit cross-legged

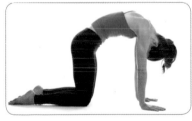

2. Cat to Cow (1 breath per movement; complete 5–8 repetitions)

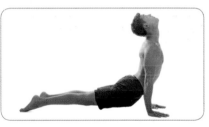

3. Sun Salutation A (1 breath per movement; perform 3 repetitions)

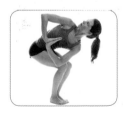

4. Thunderbolt Twist (hold for 5–8 breaths on each side)

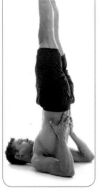

5. Shoulder Stand (hold for 8–10 breaths)

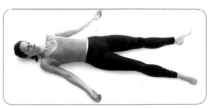

6. Corpse Pose (hold for 1 minute or longer)

STRENGTHEN AND TONE

Some beginners are surprised to learn that yoga can build muscle. There are no dumbbells here; the following sequences utilize the body's own weight to strengthen and tone. Follow these flows to cultivate well-rounded strength as you tone your upper body, lower body, and core. To enhance the strengthening benefits, simply add longer holds.

MUSCLE SEQUENCE 1

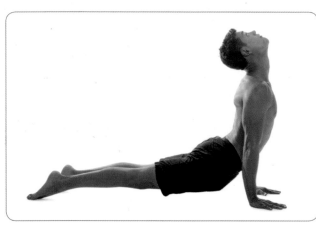

1. Sun Salutation A (perform 3 times, with 1 breath per movement)

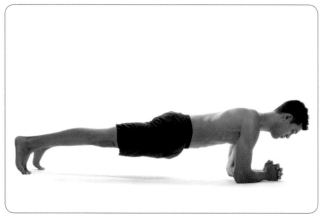

2. Forearm Plank (hold for 5–10 breaths)

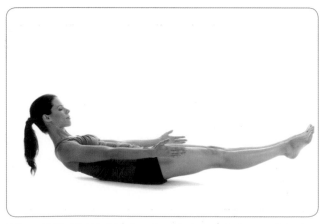

3. Boat to Half Boat (hold for 3 breaths each, moving between the two poses 5 times)

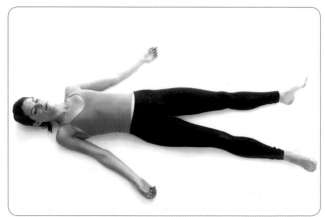

4. Corpse Pose (hold for 1 minute or longer)

MUSCLE SEQUENCE 2

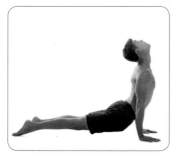

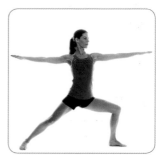

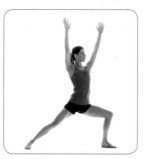

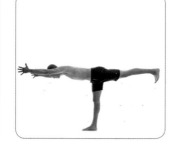

1. Sun Salutation A (perform 3 times, with 1 breath per movement)

2. Warrior I (hold for 3–5 breaths, and then repeat on the other side)

3. Warrior II (hold for 3–5 breaths, and then repeat on the other side)

4. Warrior III (hold for 3–5 breaths, and then repeat on the other side)

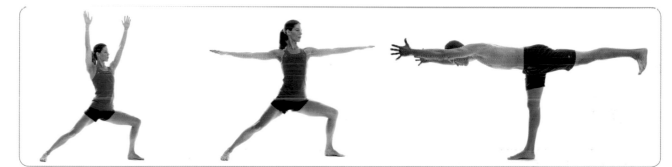

5. Move from Warrior I to II to III. Stay in each shape for one breath round (inhale/exhale) before moving on.

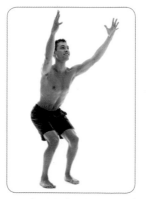

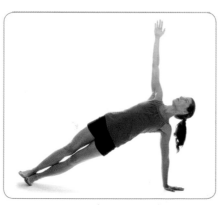

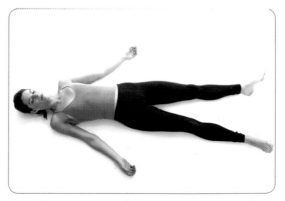

6. Chair Pose (hold for 5–8 breaths; perform 3 repetitions)

7. Side Plank (hold for 5–8 breaths, and then repeat on the other side)

8. Corpse Pose (hold for 1 breath or longer)

YOGA FIXES FOR BUSY PEOPLE

One of the amazing things about yoga is that benefits can be felt through mini-breaks and long practices alike. Below are some quick yoga breaks you can use throughout the day, whenever needed. Taking only 2 to 8 minutes, they can be used to get limber and fire up, burn a few quick calories, reduce stress, and focus your thoughts.

Feeling less than perfect is no barrier to yoga practice. Rather, it can feel great to come to the yoga mat when your body and/or emotions are in need of some repair. Think of your aches and ailments as an invitation to approach your practice from a new angle. Lower-back tension, for example, affords the opportunity to explore strengthening your spine and releasing tight muscles. When something is ailing you, you are invited to go deep: there's no room to flail around or be careless in a shape. Rather, move through these sequences deliberately—or, as we often say in yoga, "with intention."

SLEEPY NO MORE

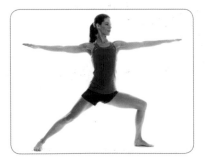

1. Child's Pose (hold for 5–8 breaths)

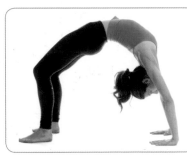

2. Mountain Pose (hold for 3–5 breaths)

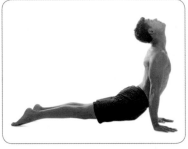

3. Sun Salutation A (hold each movement for 2–3 breaths)

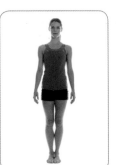

4. Warrior I (hold for 5 breaths, and then switch sides and repeat)

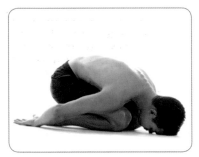

5. Warrior II (hold for 5 breaths, and then switch sides and repeat)

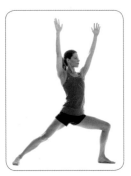

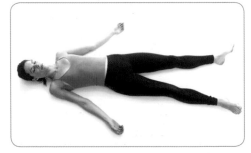

6. Full Wheel Pose (hold for 5 breaths; perform 3 repetitions)

7. Corpse Pose (take 5 deep breaths; hold for as long as needed)

FACING FEAR

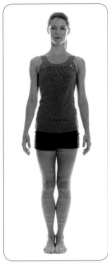

1. Mountain Pose (hold for 5–8 breaths)

2. Tree Pose (hold for 8–10 breaths, and then switch sides and repeat)

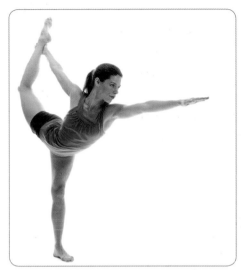

3. Dancer's Pose (hold for 8–10 breaths, and then switch sides and repeat)

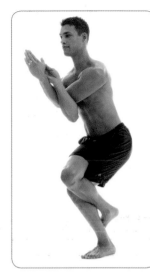

4. Eagle Pose (hold for 8–10 breaths, and then switch sides and repeat. For a balance challenge, try tipping the shape forward and then back up again)

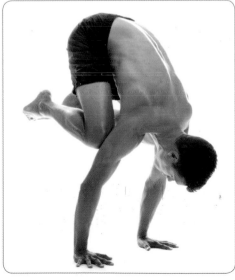

5. Crow Pose (hold for 8–10 breaths)

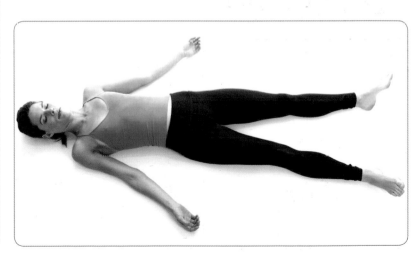

6. Corpse Pose (hold for 1 minute or longer)

LOWER-BACK TENSION RELEASE

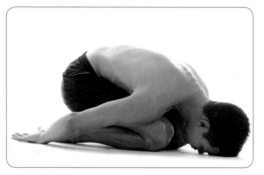

1. Child's Pose (hold for 8–10 breaths)

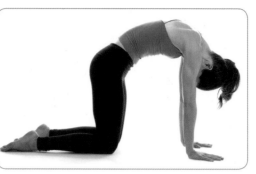

2. Cat to Cow (1 breath per movement; perform 5–8 repetitions)

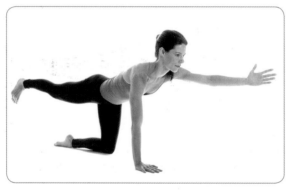

3. Spinal Arm Balance (hold for 3–5 breaths on each side)

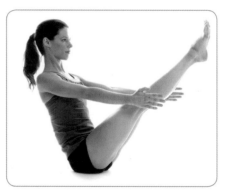

4. Boat Pose (hold for 5–8 breaths; perform 2 repetitions)

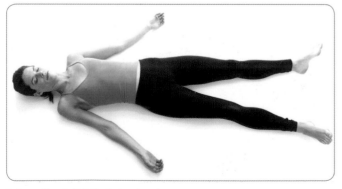

5. Corpse Pose (hold for 1 minute or longer)

STRESS BUSTER

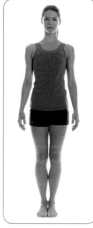

1. Mountain Pose (hold for 3–5 breaths)

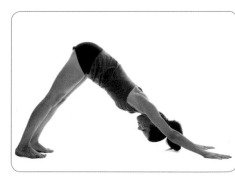

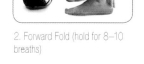

2. Forward Fold (hold for 8–10 breaths)

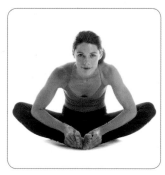

3. Butterfly Pose (hold for 8–10 breaths)

4. Downward-Facing Dog (hold for 5–8 breaths)

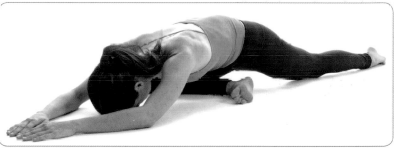

5. Pigeon Pose (move into this from Downward-Facing Dog. Stay in each side 10-15 breaths. Switch sides.)

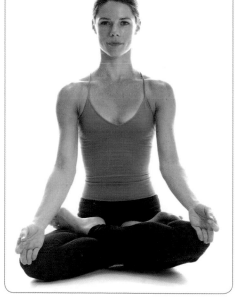

6. Full Lotus Pose (hold for 1 minute or longer)

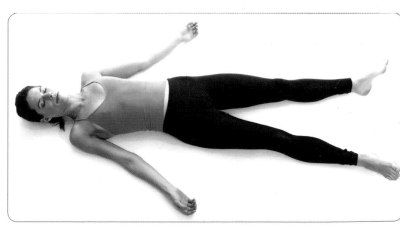

7. Corpse Pose (place one hand on your stomach and the other on your heart)

UPPER BODY BLAST

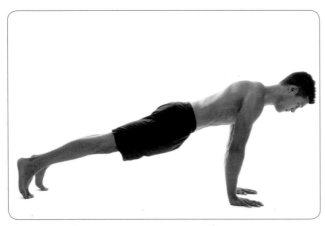

1. Plank (hold for 5 breaths, release, repeat for 8 breaths, release, then repeat for 10 breaths)

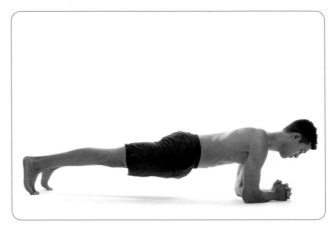

2. Forearm Plank (hold for 8 breaths)

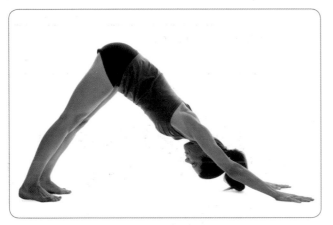

3. Downward-Facing Dog (hold for 5–8 breath)

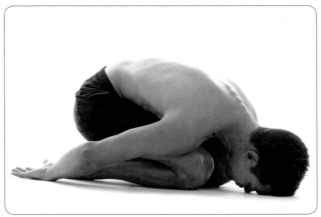

4. Child's Pose (5 or more breaths)

BELLY TONER

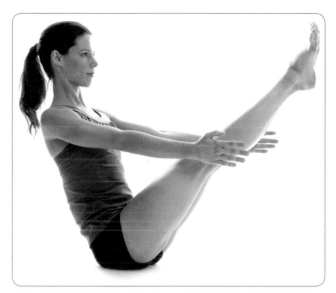

1. Boat Pose (hold for 5 breaths)

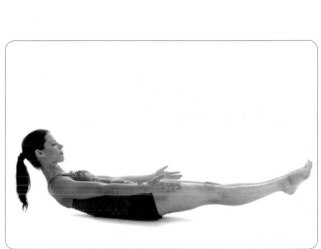

2. Boat to Half Boat (perform 5–10 repetitions)

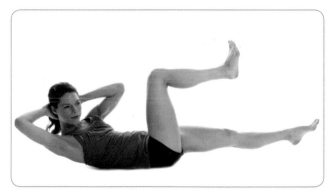

3. Yoga Bicycles (perform to a count of 10)

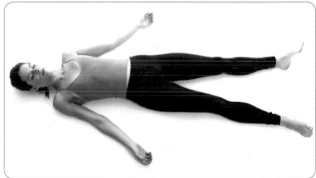

4. Corpse Pose (hold for as long as desired)

POST-WORK DECOMPRESS

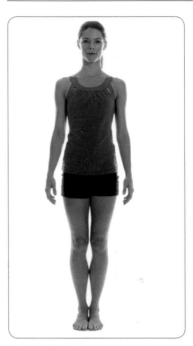

1. Mountain Pose (hold for 5–8 breaths)

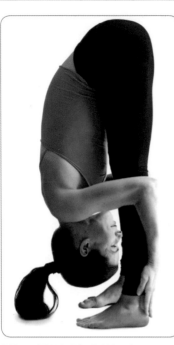

2. Forward Fold (hold for 8–10 breaths

FOOD FOR THOUGHT

"Before you've practiced, the theory is useless. After you've practiced, the theory is obvious." ~ *David Williams*

"When the breath wanders the mind also is unsteady. But when the breath is calmed the mind too will be still, and the yogi achieves long life. Therefore, one should learn to control the breath." ~ *Hatha Yoga Pradipika*

"The world is the gymnasium where we come to make ourselves strong." ~ *Swami Vivekananda*

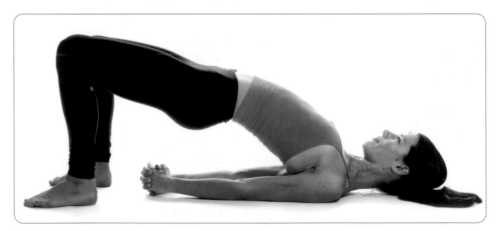

3. Bridge Pose (hold for 5 breaths)

RELAX ME NOW

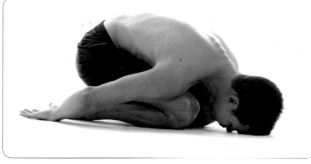

1. Child's Pose (hold for 8–10 breaths)

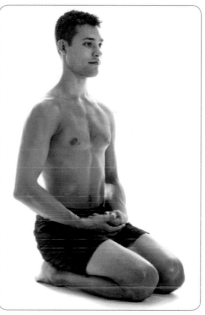

2. Hero Pose (hold for 5–8 breaths)

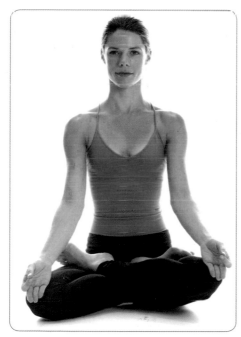

3. Full Lotus Pose (hold for 5 breaths)

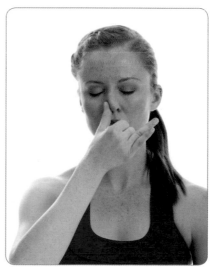

4. Alternate-Nostril Breathing (perform 5–10 rounds)

ABOUT THE AUTHOR

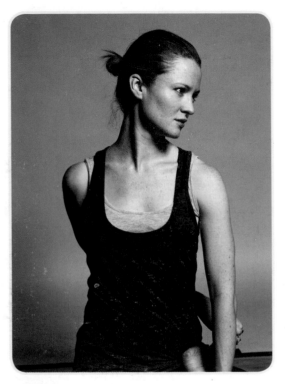

Sarah Herrington is a yoga teacher and writer living in New York City. In addition to teaching yoga in the city's public charter schools and studios, she trains and certifies new yoga teachers. Sarah draws upon more than 500 hours of training in both adult Vinyasa yoga and youth yoga, coupled with a decade of personal practice. She is the author of *OM Schooled* (Addriya, 2012), a resource for effectively teaching yoga to children, as well as a collection of poetry titled *Always Moving* (YBK Publishers, Inc./Bowery Books, 2011). A contributor to wellness site Mindbodygreen.com and various other online and print publications, Sarah believes that yoga practice can boost health, wellness, and creativity. She can be found online at www.sarahherrington.com and www.om-schooled.com.

DEDICATION: To all of my teachers, with gratitude.

ACKNOWLEDGMENTS

I'd like to thank the following amazing folks for helping make this book possible! Dori O'Brien for the wonderful support and connection, Edward Vilga for sharing insight, and Susan Kennedy for a safe haven. Thank you to Danielle Scaramuzzo for great and thoughtful design work, and to Erica Gordon-Mallin for deep dedication and exceptional editing.

Model James W. White is an instructor at Yoga to the People in New York City. He became certified to teach yoga while a college student in Boston in 2005, and in 2010 earned a 200-hour certification in Vinyasa Yoga with additional training in Traditional Hot Yoga.

Model Sara Blowers was born and raised in Los Angeles County, California. She had an on-and-off relationship with yoga before committing to a daily practice in 2010. She currently teaches at Yoga to the People in New York City, and is studying at the Dharma Yoga Center New York for a 500-hour certification.

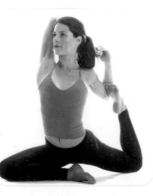